MEDITERRANEAN
DIET

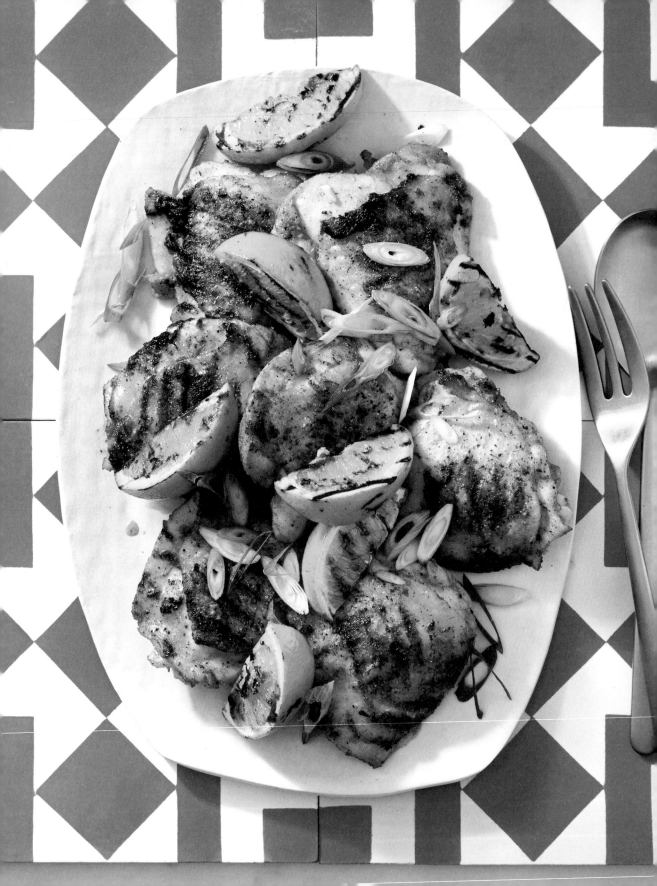

GOOD
HOUSEKEEPING

MEDITERRANEAN
DIET

70 EASY, HEALTHY RECIPES

★ GOOD FOOD GUARANTEED ★

HEARST
books

HEARSTBOOKS

An Imprint of Sterling Publishing Co., Inc.
1166 Avenue of the Americas
New York, NY 10036

ISBN 978-1-61837-294-9

The Good Housekeeping Cookbook Seal guarantees that the recipes in this publication meet the strict standards of the Good Housekeeping Institute. The Institute has been a source of reliable information and a consumer advocate since 1900 and established its seal of approval in 1909. Every recipe in this publication has been tested until perfect for ease, reliability, and great taste by the Good Housekeeping Test Kitchen.

Distributed in Canada by Sterling Publishing, Inc.
c/o Canadian Manda Group, 664 Annette Street
Toronto, Ontario M6S 2C8, Canada
Distributed in Australia by NewSouth Books
University of New South Wales, Sydney, NSW 2052, Australia

For information about custom editions, special sales, and premium and corporate purchases, please contact Sterling Special Sales at 800-805-5489 or specialsales@sterlingpublishing.com.

Manufactured in China

2 4 6 8 10 9 7 5 3 1

sterlingpublishing.com
goodhousekeeping.com

Cover design by Elizabeth Mihaltse Lindy
Interior design by Sharon Jacobs
Photography credits on page 126

Contents

FOREWORD **7**

INTRODUCTION **9**

Tapas & Small Plates 13

Soups & Salads 33

Grains, Beans & Potatoes 53

Mains 75

Meatless Meals & Vegetables 109

INDEX 124

PHOTOGRAPHY CREDITS 126

METRIC CONVERSION CHARTS 127

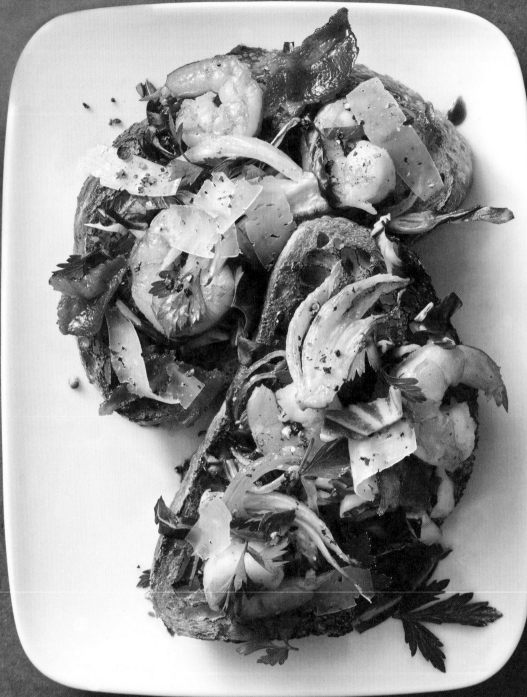

RADICCHIO SALAD WITH
ROASTED FENNEL & SHRIMP
(PAGE 48)

Foreword

If you regularly cook from *Good Housekeeping*, you're already using some of the principles of the Mediterranean diet. Although you can lose weight eating this way, I want to tell you the Mediterranean diet is not a *diet* in the calorie-reduction sense. It is a lifestyle plan that encompasses much of what you and your family love. With a focus on good-for-you fresh vegetables, fruits, grains, fish, lean meat and poultry, beans, and healthy fats, this lifestyle plan is brimming with flavor—and simple preparations for weeknight and family-friendly meals.

Do you cook mostly with olive oil or other healthy plant-based oils? Do you try to serve more fruits and vegetables? Are you cooking some vegetarian meals regularly? You've already embraced the Mediterranean diet! Eating Mediterranean is a lifestyle, so do as they do and make family dinners a time to sit around the table, relax, and catch up on the day's activities. You may notice that it helps you eat more slowly and pay more attention to the food's flavors. Plus eating more slowly will help you to know when you're full, so you'll be less prone to overeat. Jaclyn London, *Good Housekeeping*'s resident RD and nutrition guru, will explain more about the basics and benefits of eating Mediterranean-style in the introduction (page 9).

Meanwhile, if you're thinking "What about our Taco Tuesdays?", relax—the principles of the Mediterranean diet don't apply just to Mediterranean food. They work with foods from around the globe as you'll see in these pages. Whether you have time for a quick skillet meal, a sheet pan supper, or a slow-cooked stew, you'll find this book full of ideas for lunches, dinners, and snacks that will keep you satisfied. Yes, there are recipes that were developed for the slow-cooker and multi-cooker too, so you can fix it and forget it, Mediterranean-style. We've divided the book into five chapters: Tapas & Small Plates, Soups & Salads, Grains, Beans & Potatoes, Mains, and Meatless Meals & Vegetables.

You'll find riffs on favorites like Penne with Roasted Tomatoes & Spring Onion Pesto (page 65), Lemon-Dill Chicken Meatball Soup (page 39), and Feta-Dill Greek Caesar (page 49), to name a few. If you've never made Homemade Hummus (page 25) with dried chickpeas, prepare to be wowed. Occasional desserts are fine, just remember they are a treat, not a daily right.

All of these recipes have been tested until perfect and include complete nutritional information so you can plan your meals and snacks—and enjoy every bite.

SUSAN WESTMORELAND
Culinary Director, *Good Housekeeping*

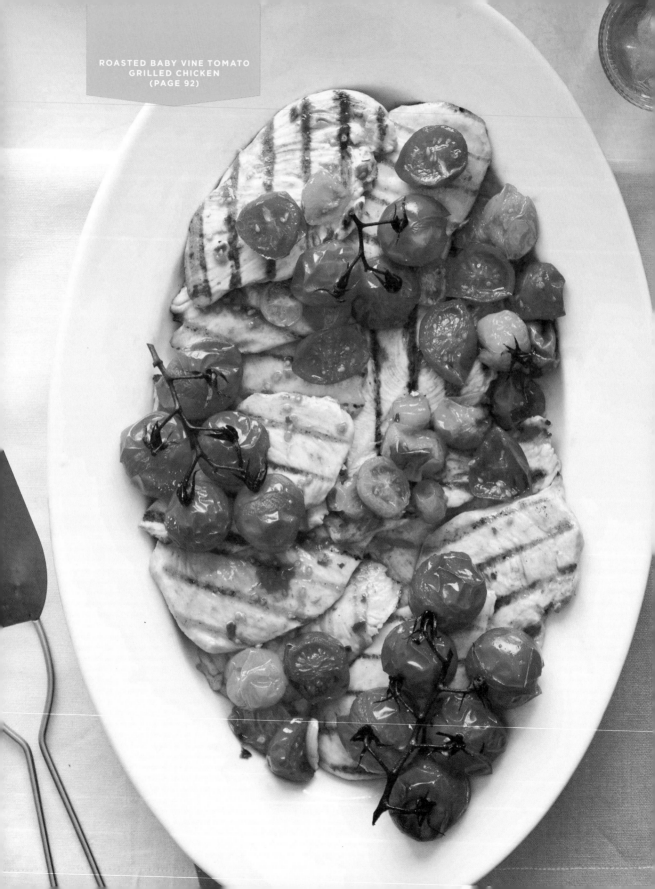

ROASTED BABY VINE TOMATO
GRILLED CHICKEN
(PAGE 92)

Introduction

Welcome to your new favorite cookbook! The Mediterranean diet has served as inspiration for centuries, and its health benefits are innumerable. This book is packed with countless recipes that aim to satisfy, and it promotes flavorful ingredients that make every meal you enjoy feel unique—without additional hassle or prep/cook time. As this style of eating is considered one of the most beneficial in the world, we're thrilled to bring a little bit of the Mediterranean cuisine and lifestyle into your home.

IS THIS A WEIGHT-LOSS DIET?

No, but it can be! But then again, so can any eating plan, so long as you're eating fewer calories than you burn.

That being said, don't let the word *diet* throw you off—Mediterranean cuisine is beneficial for your health, weight, and, most of all, your taste buds! The plan is packed with flavor and inspired by cuisine staples and regional specialties of Mediterranean countries. On this eating plan, all of your meals and snacks will prioritize plant-based ingredients, like filling, nutrient-dense veggies and fruit; high quality herbs and spices; 100% whole grains, plus legumes, nuts, and seeds. You'll also eat immune-boosting, heart-healthy seafood, plus lean cuts of beef and poultry. When eating the Mediterranean way, you'll prioritize real, whole foods and limit added sugars and saturated fats from more processed ones. These recipes also use mostly unsaturated fats from plant-based oils (especially extra-virgin olive oil) to replace butter—one of the key components of the diet that's been linked to reducing risk of chronic disease.

WHAT MAKES THE MEDITERRANEAN DIET SO GREAT?

A universal truth of the Mediterranean diet is that it's a lifestyle above all else. When eating the Mediterranean way, you are encouraged to enjoy meals with friends and loved ones; savor each flavor and indulge in delicious, quality items (like dessert and flavorful cheeses); and make time for plenty of physical activity.

IS THERE A CALORIE LIMIT OR MEAL-PLAN INVOLVED?

Nope! For that reason alone, this diet is right for everyone—and the recipes on these pages can help you make healthier, happier choices for the long-term. With that in mind: think of indulgences as add-ons instead of calorie-counting each bite—this will help you stay mindful as you eat. It'll also make it easier to cut back on sodium, saturated fat, and added sugar.

PRIORITIZE GOOD-FOR-YOU FATS

Plant-based oils are made from mostly unsaturated fats, which have been linked to lowering LDL (your "bad" cholesterol) when used to replace the mostly saturated fats you'll find in the traditional Western diet. Some of the oils you'll learn to love are canola, sesame, peanut, extra-virgin olive, flax, and hempseed oils, plus other nut-derived oils that add flavor and a slew of health benefits.

Another reason to get on the Mediterranean bandwagon? Plant-based oils are filled with polyphenolic compounds, a type of powerful antioxidant that's been linked to longevity as well as reducing the risk of diseases including heart disease, diabetes, and some cancers. These antioxidants (and other compounds derived from plants) can help to enhance nitric oxide production, which can improve vascular function by promoting blood flow to your tissues. They have also been linked to lowering blood pressure.

Another immune-boosting cuisine staple? Nuts and seeds (like almonds, peanuts, cashews, walnuts, and macadamia nuts, plus chia, flax, hemp, and sesame seeds) plus pulse-crops like chickpeas, lentils, beans and peas (and their derivatives, like chickpea flour, hummus, and tahini) are flavorful, satisfying and filling! This power-packed combination of fiber, protein and antioxidants have been linked to reduced disease risk and lowering your risk of cognitive decline. Plus, the vitamin E found in extra-virgin olive-oil (and olives of the region!) and omega-3 fatty acids may help to boost cognition and reduce risk of cognitive decline too.

EAT MORE SEAFOOD

The omega-3s found in fatty fish (like salmon, tuna, sardines, herring, and trout) and crustaceans and mollusks (shrimp, scallops, mussels, and langostines) have been proven to reduce your risk of chronic diseases and boost cognition. Plus, since omega-3s are more difficult to find in food sources, eating seafood regularly is an easy, delicious, and nutritious way to add extra health benefits from filling, flavorful fare. Seafood also has anti-inflammatory benefits.

FILL UP ON NUTRIENT-PACKED PRODUCE.

Always at the core of any health-promoting plan is delicious, nutrient-packed produce. The Mediterranean diet is no exception. On this plan, vegetables are made more prominent on the plate by giving them a starring role in all your meals. You'll eat seasonal produce roasted, sautéed, steamed, and as a flavor-booster on top of pizza, pasta, and whole grains. Fruit will also be a mainstay, providing filling fiber and immune-protective antioxidants.

CHOOSE 100% WHOLE-GRAINS

Another component of Mediterranean eating is filling, B-vitamin-packed whole grains. Delicious options include farro, buckwheat, bulgur, 100% whole-grain wheat, oats, and sorghum. These ingredients deliver key minerals we need for heart health and neurological functions.

Another Mediterranean tenant? *Mangia la pasta!* Don't skimp on this classic but rather include a higher ratio of vegetables to starches. Halve your regular pasta portions and cook pasta al dente for a better blood sugar response. Plus additional veggies and legumes will help you stay satisfied.

ENJOY CONSCIOUS INDULGENCES

The beauty of the Mediterranean diet is that it's inclusive. That said, moderation is encouraged. When choosing indulgences, make sure to stay clear of ultra-processed foods and concentrated sugars like those in beverages. (Stay hydrated with water, still or sparkling, and even consider fruit-infused H2O!)

Heavier items like decadent cheeses, processed and red meats, and sweets can be enjoyed regularly but in smaller portion sizes. By prioritizing quality over quantity, the diet tenets encourage you to be selective with added sugar and saturated fat. Plus, since you will be eating flavorful, filling meals, you will often find you don't need more than a few bites.

Additionally, there's no need to skip your morning cup of coffee or tea. Research has linked these beverages (in unsweetened form!) to heart health and immune benefits. Enjoy 300 to 400 milligrams of caffeine per day (that's about 3 or 4 8-ounce cups of coffee). And don't forget wine! The Mediterranean diet allows for a glass of wine daily (two glasses for men!).

As a lifestyle-focused eating plan, the Mediterranean diet makes the experience of a meal extra special—so gather your gang and get ready for simple, easy, and nutrient-dense meals that satisfy!

JACLYN R. LONDON, M.S., R.D., C.D.N.
Nutrition Director, Good Housekeeping Institute

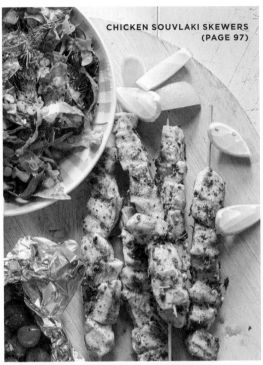

CHICKEN SOUVLAKI SKEWERS
(PAGE 97)

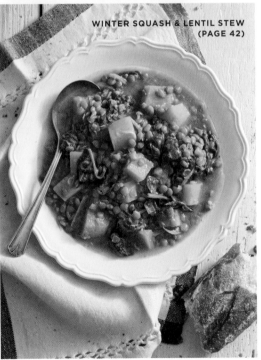

WINTER SQUASH & LENTIL STEW
(PAGE 42)

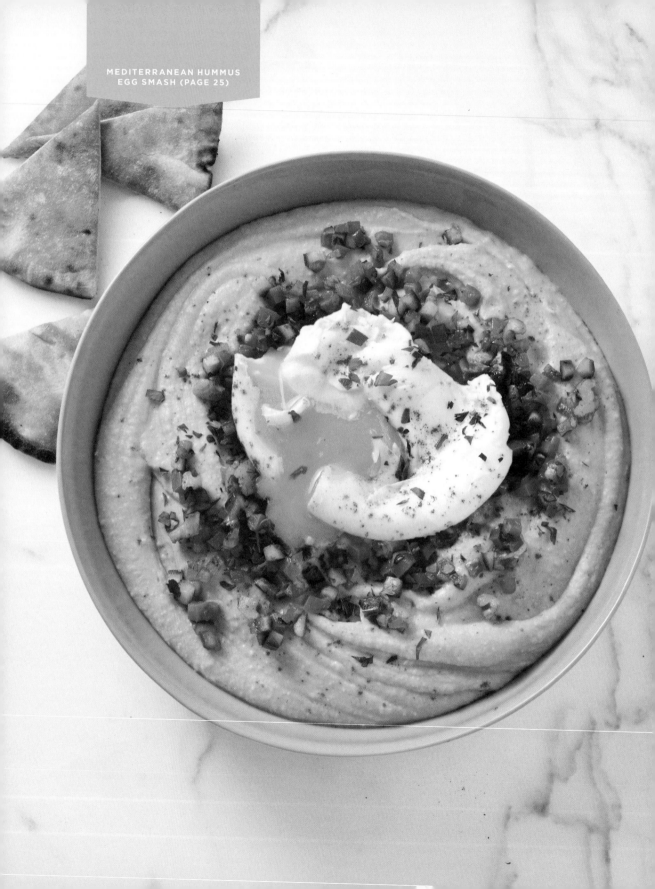

MEDITERRANEAN HUMMUS
EGG SMASH (PAGE 25)

I | Tapas & Small Plates

These dishes are made to share before a main meal or as a midday snack. Versatile and colorful dips and spreads can be served with whole-grain crackers or fresh seasonal vegetables. Not sure what to make for your next dinner party? Offer a variety of these dishes as *tapas*, or small, savory dishes usually served with drinks. Kebabs, flatbreads, and other small plates will satisfy everyone at the table!

Spicy Italian Mussels & "Frites" 15

Grilled Leek, Zucchini & Ricotta Pizza 17

Greek Yellow Split Pea Dip 18

Arugula Pesto Crostini 19

Cherry Tomato Confit 21

Old Bay Peel 'n' Eat Shrimp 23

Swordfish Kebabs with Mint Pesto 24

Mediterranean Hummus Egg Smash 25

Crispy Cod Cakes with Almond-Pepper Vinaigrette 27

Roasted Artichokes with Caesar Dip 29

Plum Tomato & Eggplant Shakshuka 31

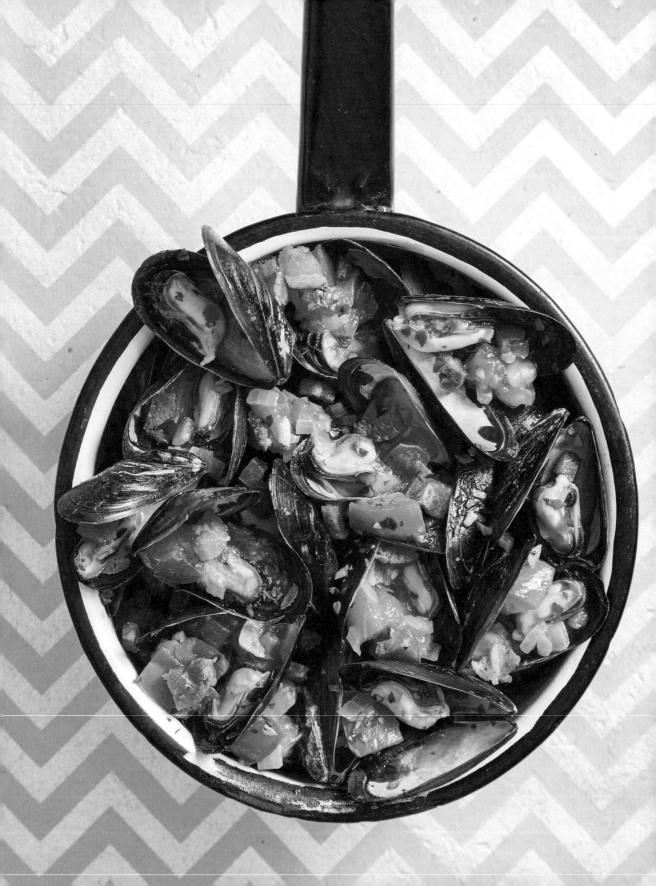

Spicy Italian Mussels & "Frites"

French fries soak up the spicy tomato sauce perfectly.
Consider baking them for a healthier alternative.

PREP: **10 MINUTES**   TOTAL: **40 MINUTES**

12 ounces frozen french fries

2 ounces pancetta, chopped

1 tablespoon olive oil

1 small onion, chopped

2 cloves garlic, chopped

¾ teaspoon crushed red pepper

2 tomatoes, chopped

2 pounds mussels, scrubbed and debearded

3 tablespoons grated Parmesan cheese

Chopped fresh parsley, for garnish

1. Cook the french fries as the label directs.

2. Meanwhile, in an 8-quart saucepot, cook the pancetta in the olive oil on medium heat until crisp, about 6 minutes, stirring often. With a slotted spoon, transfer the pancetta to a plate. To the pot, add the onion, garlic, and crushed red pepper. Cook 4 minutes, stirring often. Add the tomatoes. Increate the heat to high and bring to a simmer.

3. Add the mussels, reduce the heat to medium, and cover the pot. Cook until the mussels open, 4 to 7 minutes, stirring twice.

4. Toss the hot fries with the Parmesan; serve the fries alongside the mussels, garnished with pancetta and parsley.

SERVES 4: About 335 calories, 25g protein, 28g carbohydrates, 16g fat (4g saturated), 3g fiber, 660mg sodium.

TIP

Scrub mussels well under cold running water. To debeard, grasp the hairlike beard firmly with your thumb and forefinger and pull it away, or scrap it off with a knife. That said, cultivated mussels usually do not have beards.

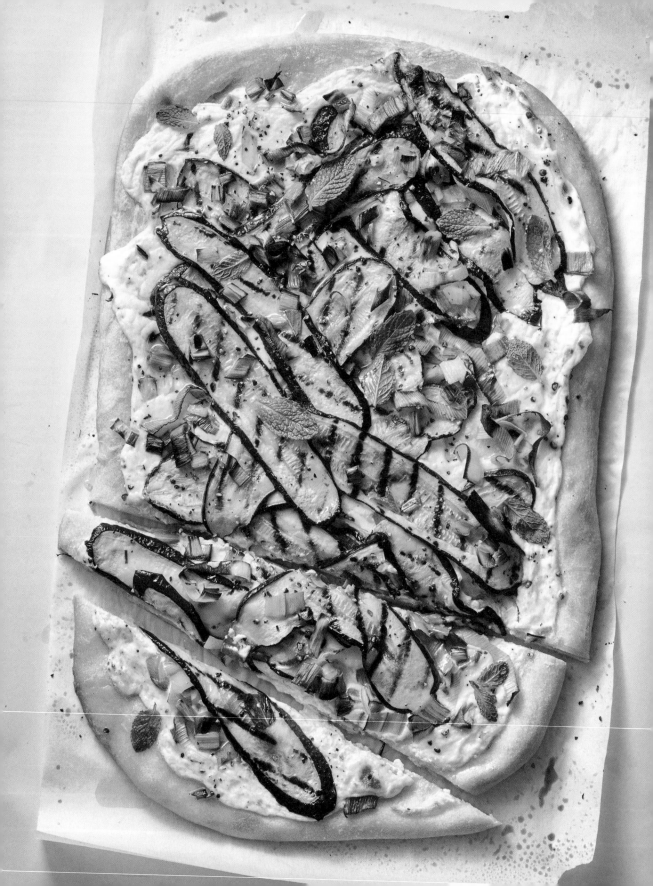

Grilled Leek, Zucchini & Ricotta Pizza

This rich flatbread will be the perfect appetizer
at your next dinner party.

PREP: **15 MINUTES**   TOTAL: **45 MINUTES**

1 pound whole-grain pizza dough

1 large leek

Olive oil

Kosher salt and ground black pepper

2 large zucchini

1 lemon

2 cups ricotta cheese

**Extra-virgin olive oil and fresh mint,
    for topping (optional)**

1. Preheat the oven to 425°F. Line a rimmed baking sheet with parchment paper.

2. Place the pizza dough on the prepared baking sheet and shape it into a large rectangle. Bake for 10 minutes. Set the baking sheet and crust aside and increase the oven temperature to 475°F.

3. Meanwhile, preheat the grill to medium-high. Halve the leek lengthwise, brush the cut sides of each half with oil, and season with salt and pepper. Slice the zucchini lengthwise, brush with oil, and season with salt and pepper. Grill the leek and zucchini until tender, 5 to 8 minutes. Thinly slice the leek crosswise. Place the grilled vegetables in a bowl.

4. From the lemon, finely grate 2 teaspoons zest and set aside; squeeze 3 tablespoons lemon juice. Toss the grilled vegetables with the lemon juice.

5. In a separate bowl, mix the ricotta with the lemon zest and ½ teaspoon salt; spread it evenly on the baked crust. Top with the grilled vegetables. Bake until browned, 5 to 8 minutes. Top with extra-virgin olive oil and mint, if desired.

SERVES 4: About 575 calories, 22g protein, 60g carbohydrates, 27g fat (12g saturated), 4g fiber, 1,235mg sodium.

Greek Yellow Split Pea Dip

Serve this creamy dip with crunchy whole-grain crackers or your favorite crudités for a satisfying combination of textures and flavors.

1 cup dried yellow split peas

2½ cups water

1 small onion, finely chopped

1 large clove garlic, crushed
   with a garlic press

1 bay leaf

½ teaspoon ground turmeric

Kosher salt

2 tablespoons extra-virgin olive oil,
   plus more for serving

1 tablespoon fresh lemon juice

Finely chopped red onion, finely chopped
   fresh parsley, and paprika, for serving
   (optional)

1. In a small saucepan, combine the split peas with the water and bring to a boil, skimming any foam that rises to the surface. Lower the heat and add the onion, garlic, bay leaf, turmeric, and ½ teaspoon salt; simmer until the split peas are very tender, 50 to 60 minutes.

2. Discard the bay leaf and transfer the mixture and any remaining liquid to a food processor. Add the olive oil and lemon juice and process until smooth.

3. Transfer the dip to a serving bowl and top with red onion, parsley, and a sprinkle of paprika, if desired.

SERVES 8: About 130 calories, 6g protein, 18g carbohydrates, 5g fat (1g saturated), 7g fiber, 120mg sodium.

Arugula Pesto Crostini

Sneak even more greens into this flavorful pesto spread.
It's delicious as a topping on a crostini.

TOTAL: **5 MINUTES**

2 cups baby arugula

⅓ cup grated Parmesan cheese

¼ cup pine nuts, toasted

1 tablespoon fresh lemon juice

1 clove garlic

½ cup extra-virgin olive oil

Kosher salt

¾ cup ricotta cheese

1 whole-grain baguette, cut into 1-inch slices, toasted

Pine nuts and lemon zest, for serving

1. In a food processor, pulse the arugula, Parmesan, pine nuts, lemon juice, garlic, olive oil, and ¼ teaspoon salt until smooth. Makes ¾ cups. Store in the refrigerator for 3 days.

2. To serve, spread ricotta onto the toasted bread slices, top with about 1 tablespoon of the pesto, a few pine nuts, and lemon zest.

SERVES 12: About 200 calories, 4g protein, 8g carbohydrates, 17g fat (4g saturated), 0g fiber, 220mg sodium.

> **TIP**
>
> This pesto would also make a great sauce for a cold pasta salad or a marinade for chicken.

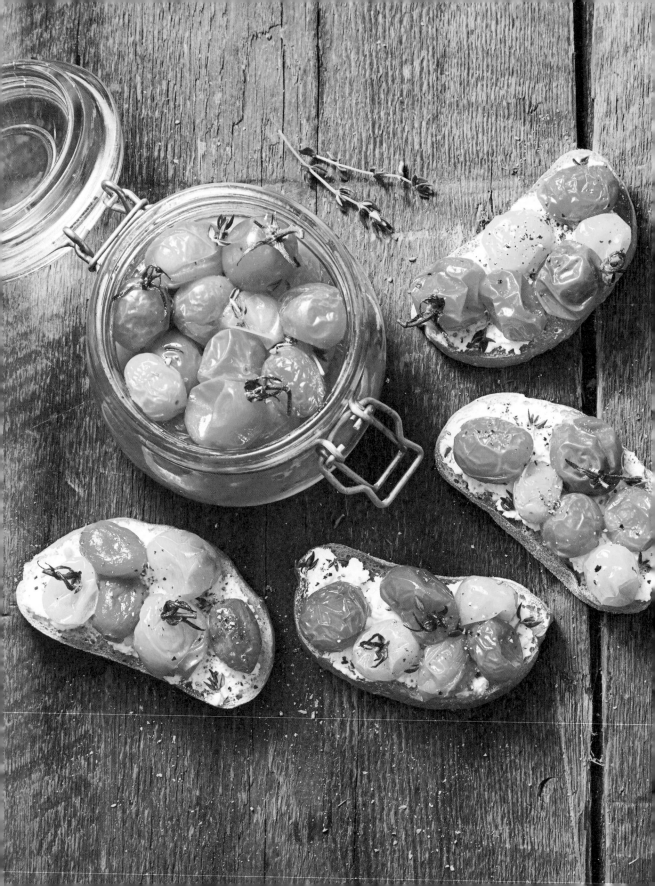

Cherry Tomato Confit

This four-main-ingredient confit dresses up your
cocktail hour's crostini and bruschetta.

PREP: 10 MINUTES TOTAL: 1 HOUR

4 pints cherry tomatoes

6 cloves garlic, smashed and peeled

6 sprigs fresh thyme

¼ cup extra-virgin olive oil

Salt and ground black pepper

1. Preheat the oven to 350°F.

2. On a large rimmed baking sheet, toss the cherry tomatoes, garlic, and thyme with the olive oil and ¼ teaspoon each salt and pepper.

3. Bake until the tomatoes are wrinkled and fragrant, 45 to 50 minutes, shaking the baking sheet halfway through. Remove from the oven and let cool.

4. Use the confit on bruschetta, in salads, or over pasta, grilled meat, or fish. To store, transfer the confit to a jar, top with olive oil to cover, and refrigerate for up to 1 week. Makes 4 cups.

SERVES 16 (¼ cup each): About 45 calories, 1g protein, 3g carbohydrates, 4g fat (1g saturated), 1g fiber, 35mg sodium.

TIP

Confit comes from the French word *confire*, which means "to preserve."

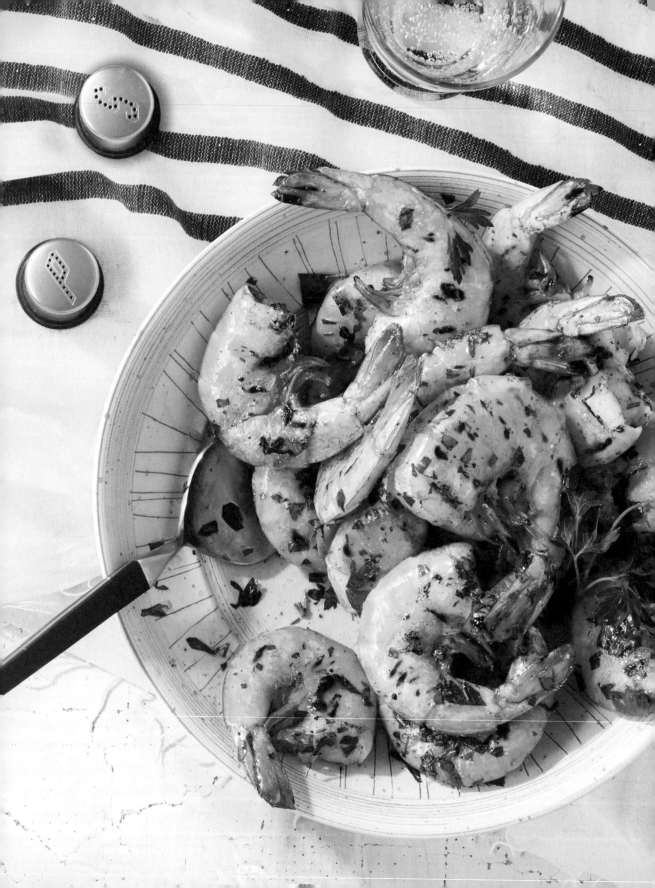

Old Bay Peel 'n' Eat Shrimp

These seasoned shrimp are a great appetizer for
a crowd willing to get a little messy.

PREP: **5 MINUTES**   TOTAL: **10 MINUTES**

**1½ pounds shell-on deveined
large (16- to 20-count) shrimp**

1 tablespoon olive oil

3 teaspoons Old Bay seasoning

¼ cup chopped fresh parsley

1. Prepare outdoor grill for direct grilling over high heat.

2. Toss shrimp with olive oil and 1½ teaspoons Old Bay seasoning.

3. Thread shrimp onto skewers and grill 3 to 5 minutes, turning over once, until opaque.

4. Remove shrimp from skewers and transfer to a large bowl. Sprinkle with parsley and 1½ teaspoons Old Bay seasoning; toss to combine. Serve immediately.

SERVES 4: About 160 calories, 27g protein, 0g carbohydrates, 5g fat (1g saturated), 0g fiber, 790mg sodium.

TIP

Got leftovers? Toss these shrimp on a salad the next day.

Swordfish Kebabs with Mint Pesto

Thanks to a mint, parsley, and lemon marinade, grilled cubes of swordfish pack a dose of refreshing flavor.

PREP: **10 MINUTES**   TOTAL: **25 MINUTES**

¼ cup sliced almonds

1 large clove garlic, smashed

1 cup packed fresh mint leaves

¼ cup packed fresh parsley leaves

1 tablespoon grated lemon zest (from 1 medium lemon)

5 tablespoons extra-virgin olive oil

Salt and ground black pepper

Pinch of crushed red pepper (optional)

1½ pounds thick-cut swordfish steaks, cut into 1½-inch cubes

1. If you're using bamboo skewers, soak them for at least 30 minutes in warm water.

2. Make the mint pesto. In a food processor, pulse the almonds and garlic until finely chopped. Add the mint, parsley, and lemon zest; pulse until finely ground, stopping and scraping the bowl occasionally. Transfer the mixture to a medium bowl; stir in the olive oil, ½ teaspoon salt, ¼ teaspoon black pepper, and crushed red pepper, if using.

3. In another medium bowl, combine the swordfish with one-third of the pesto, tossing to combine. Refrigerate for at least 30 minutes or up to 4 hours.

4. Preheat the grill to medium-high. Thread 3 pieces of swordfish onto each skewer. Grill the kebabs until cooked through, 2 to 3 minutes on each side. Serve with the remaining pesto.

SERVES 4: About 420 calories, 31g protein, 4g carbohydrates, 30g fat (5g saturated), 3g fiber, 420mg sodium.

TIP

When choosing a fish to grill, make sure it has a firm and meaty texture, like swordfish.

Mediterranean Hummus Egg Smash

This homemade hummus recipe, topped with a soft poached egg, is the stunner of the brunch table. See photo on page 12.

PREP: 15 MINUTES   TOTAL: 30 MINUTES

1 tablespoon olive oil

1 small red bell pepper, seeded and finely chopped

1 small red onion, finely chopped

½ teaspoon smoked paprika, plus more for garnish

Salt

1 mini cucumber, finely chopped

¼ cup finely chopped walnuts

2 tablespoons finely chopped fresh parsley

1 tablespoon distilled white vinegar

1 large egg

2 cups store-bought or homemade hummus

Whole-grain pitas, for serving

1. In a 10-inch skillet, heat the olive oil on medium. Add the bell pepper, onion, paprika, and ¼ teaspoon salt; cook until the vegetables are tender, 6 to 8 minutes, stirring occasionally. Cool slightly, then stir in the cucumber, walnuts, and parsley.

2. In a deep 10-inch skillet, heat the vinegar and 1 inch of cold water to simmering on medium heat. Crack the egg into a small cup. Gently swirl the water in a circular motion and place the egg into it; stir the water gently to gather the egg white around the yolk. Cook until the white is set but the yolk is still runny, 3 to 5 minutes.

3. Meanwhile, spread the hummus in a shallow bowl; top with the vegetable mixture, creating an indentation in the center. When the egg is cooked, remove it from the water with slotted spoon and gently blot it dry on a paper towel before placing it in the indentation. Garnish with a pinch of paprika. Serve immediately with the warm pitas.

SERVES 8: About 305 calories, 11g protein, 26g carbohydrates, 20g fat (2g saturated), 8g fiber, 357mg sodium.

HOMEMADE HUMMUS

In a 4-quart saucepan, combine **1 cup dried chickpeas** and **1 teaspoon baking soda** with **cold water** to cover by 2 inches. Let soak overnight. Drain (do not rinse); return the chickpeas to the saucepan along with cold water to cover by 2 inches. Heat to boiling on high. Reduce the heat to medium and simmer until the chickpeas are soft and the skins have loosened, about 1 hour. In a food processor, pulse **4 cloves garlic**, **6 tablespoons fresh lemon juice**, **¾ teaspoon salt**, and **¾ teaspoon ground cumin** until combined. Add **¾ cup tahini** (sesame paste) and **⅓ cup water**; pulse until smooth. Drain the chickpeas and add to the tahini mixture; process until smooth, stopping and stirring occasionally. Transfer hummus to an airtight container and refrigerate up to 2 weeks. Makes about 3½ cups.

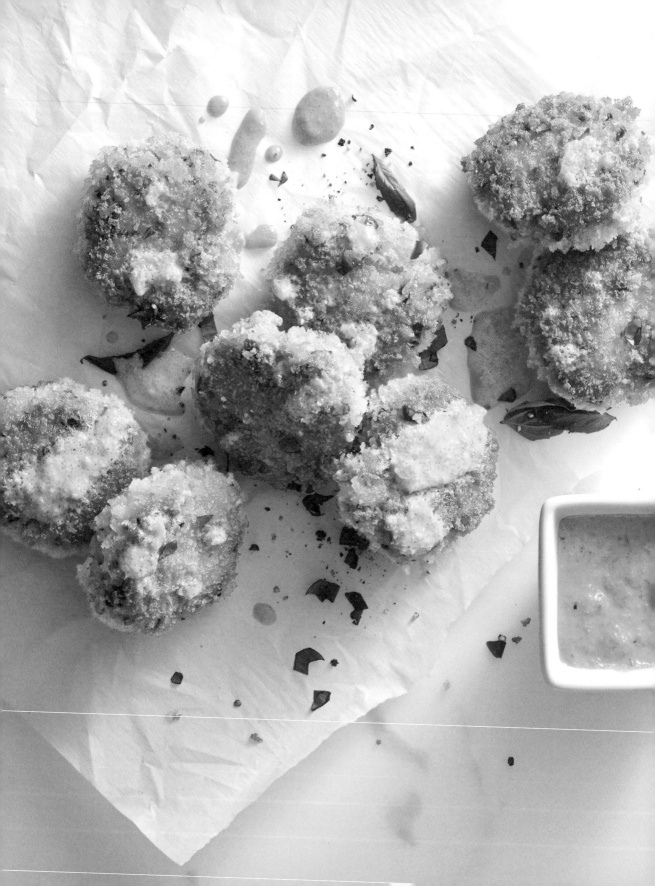

Crispy Cod Cakes with Almond-Pepper Vinaigrette

These cod poppers make the perfect appetizer when served over
a bed of salad greens and topped with a savory vinaigrette.

PREP: 15 MINUTES **TOTAL: 20 MINUTES**

⅓ cup salted almonds

5 tablespoons sherry vinegar

5 tablespoons extra-virgin olive oil

Salt

⅓ cup roasted red peppers

1 pound cod fillets, cut into chunks

⅓ cup fresh basil leaves, packed

3 cloves garlic, crushed with
   a garlic press

½ teaspoon smoked paprika

Ground black pepper

1 large egg, beaten

1 cup whole wheat panko

2 tablespoons vegetable oil

Salad greens, for serving

1. Make the almond-pepper vinaigrette: In a
blender, puree the almonds, vinegar, olive oil,
and ¼ teaspoon salt until smooth. Add the
roasted red peppers; pulse until almost smooth.
Set aside.

2. In a food processor, pulse the fish fillets, basil,
garlic, smoked paprika, and ¼ teaspoon each
salt and pepper until the fish is finely chopped,
stirring occasionally. Form the mixture into
8 patties; dip each into the egg and then the
panko, patting it to adhere.

3. In a 12-inch skillet, heat the vegetable oil on
medium; panfry the fish cakes until they are
a deep golden brown, 3 minutes per side.

4. Serve the cod cakes with the vinaigrette
and salad greens.

SERVES 4: About 450 calories, 24g protein,
21g carbohydrates, 30g fat (4g saturated),
3g fiber, 470mg sodium.

TIP

Haddock can be substituted for cod in this
recipe, if desired.

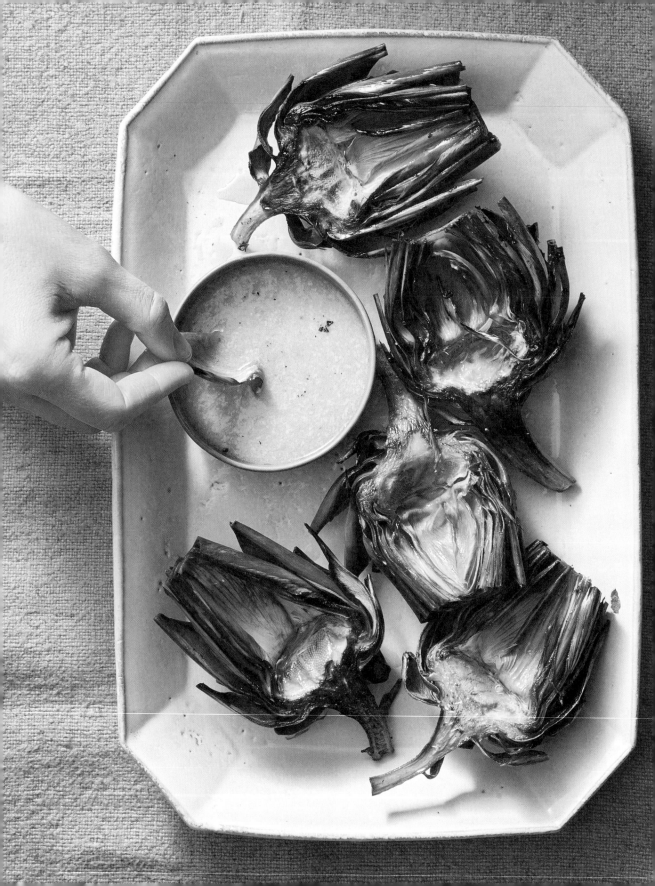

Roasted Artichokes with Caesar Dip

Just wait until you try the cheesy mustard sauce.

PREP: 45 MINUTES   TOTAL: 1 HOUR 20 MINUTES

3 globe artichokes

2 lemons

4 tablespoons olive oil

Kosher salt

1 small clove garlic, crushed with a garlic press

1 teaspoon Dijon mustard

½ teaspoon Worcestershire sauce

¼ cup grated Parmesan cheese

1. Preheat the oven to 425°F. Line a rimmed baking sheet with aluminum foil.

2. Rinse the artichokes and dry them with paper towels. Trim the stems and cut ¼ inch off the top of each. Use kitchen shears to cut off the tip of each leaf. Use your hands to pull and loosen the leaves to open up the artichokes. Slice the artichokes in half vertically and use a small knife to cut out the fuzzy centers and purple leaves.

3. Place the artichoke halves on the prepared baking sheet. Squeeze the juice from half of lemon on the cut sides of the artichokes and rub the squeezed lemon half over each artichoke half. Drizzle with 1 tablespoon of the olive oil and season with ¼ teaspoon salt. Flip the artichokes over and repeat with another lemon half, 1 tablespoon of the olive oil, and ¼ teaspoon salt.

4. Arrange the artichokes, cut sides down, on the prepared baking sheet, cover with foil, and roast until golden brown and tender, 35 to 40 minutes.

5. Meanwhile, sprinkle ¼ teaspoon salt over the crushed garlic; using a large knife, rub and scrape the salt into the garlic to make a paste. Transfer to a bowl.

6. Finely grate the zest from the remaining lemon into the bowl, then squeeze the juice into the bowl of garlic (you should have at least 3 tablespoons of juice). Whisk in the mustard, Worcestershire sauce, and the remaining 2 tablespoons olive oil. Stir in the Parmesan. Serve with artichokes for dipping.

SERVES 6: About 135 calories, 4g protein, 9g carbohydrates, 11g fat (2g saturated), 4g fiber, 410mg sodium.

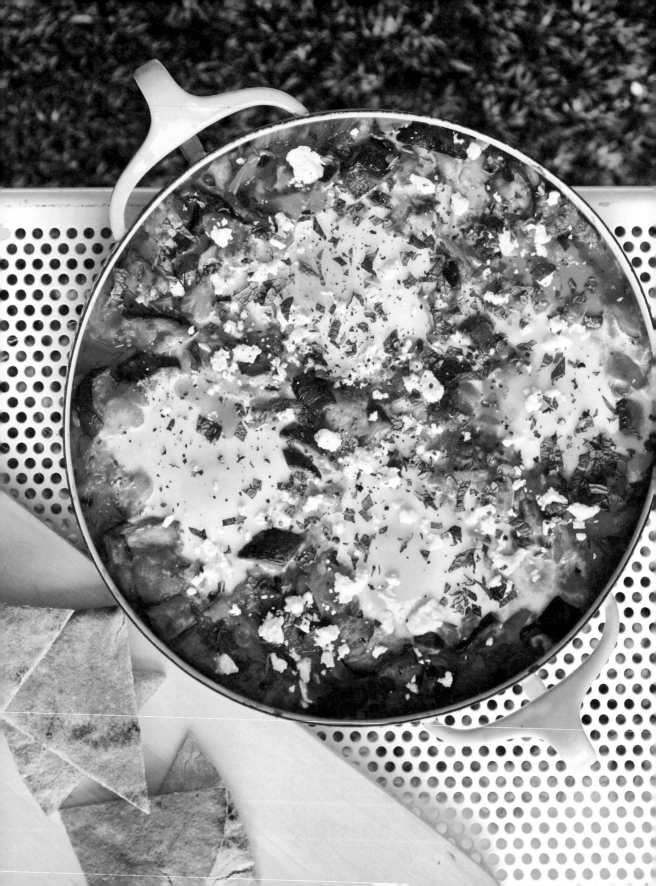

Plum Tomato & Eggplant Shakshuka

You're going to want to get extra pita for scooping up this eggy goodness.

PREP: 25 MINUTES   TOTAL: 1 HOUR 25 MINUTES

2 eggplants (about 2 pounds), trimmed and sliced into ¾-inch-thick rounds

3½ tablespoons olive oil

Kosher salt

¼ cup chopped fresh mint

1 white onion, coarsely chopped

3 cloves garlic, sliced

2 teaspoons hot paprika

1 teaspoon ground cumin

¼ teaspoon crushed red pepper

5 ripe tomatoes (about 1¾ pounds), chopped, juices reserved

½ cup tomato puree

Ground black pepper

4 large eggs

2 ounces feta cheese, crumbled (½ cup)

2 whole wheat pitas, halved and toasted (optional)

1. Preheat the oven to 375°F. On a rimmed baking sheet, brush the cut sides of the eggplant with 1½ tablespoons of the olive oil and season with ¼ teaspoon salt. Roast until soft and golden, about 25 minutes, turning once halfway through. Coarsely chop the eggplant and toss it in a bowl with 2 tablespoons of the mint.

2. Increase the oven temperature to 425°F. In a large ovenproof skillet, heat the remaining 2 tablespoons olive oil on medium. Add the onion and garlic; cook, stirring, until beginning to brown on the edges, about 8 minutes.

3. Stir in the paprika, cumin, and crushed red pepper. Cook, stirring, for 1 minute. Add the tomatoes with their juices and the tomato puree; cook until the tomatoes break down, stirring occasionally, about 15 minutes. Add the eggplant; cook 2 minutes. Stir in ½ teaspoon salt and ¼ teaspoon black pepper.

4. Remove the skillet from the heat. With a spoon, create 4 indentations in the sauce; crack the eggs, placing one in each indentation. Transfer the pan to the oven. Cook until the egg whites are set but the yolks are still runny, 5 to 7 minutes. Top with feta and the remaining mint. Serve with toasted pitas, if desired.

SERVES 4: About 365 calories, 14g protein, 35g carbohydrates, 21g fat (6g saturated), 12g fiber, 645mg sodium.

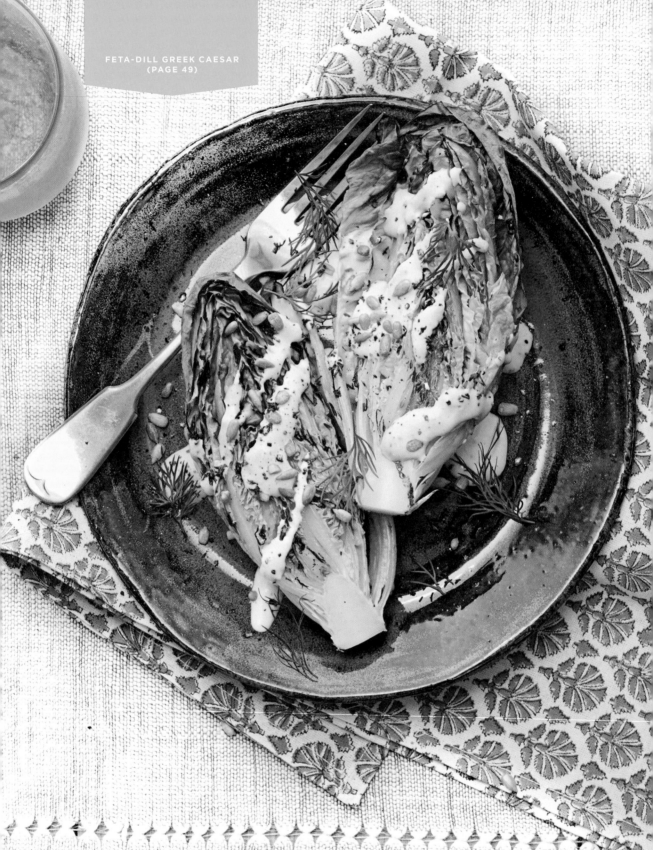

FETA-DILL GREEK CAESAR
(PAGE 49)

2 | Soups & Salads

From unique dishes to classics with a twist, this section includes soups and salads for every season. Warm stews and hearty roasted mixtures are perfect for colder months, while bright vegetable purees and fresh leafy salads satisfy in the spring and summer. Offering lots of options, these recipes are tasty as appetizers, entrées, or side dishes.

Spring Minestrone 35

Butternut Squash & White
Bean Soup 37

Cauliflower Soup 38

Lemon-Dill Chicken
Meatball Soup 39

Smoky Vegan Black Bean Soup 41

Winter Squash & Lentil Stew 42

Mixed Greens & Herb Toss Salad 43

Beet, Mushroom & Avocado Salad .. 45

Green Goddess Carrot Salad 47

Radicchio Salad with Roasted
Fennel & Shrimp 48

Feta-Dill Greek Caesar 49

Kale & Roasted Cauliflower Salad ... 51

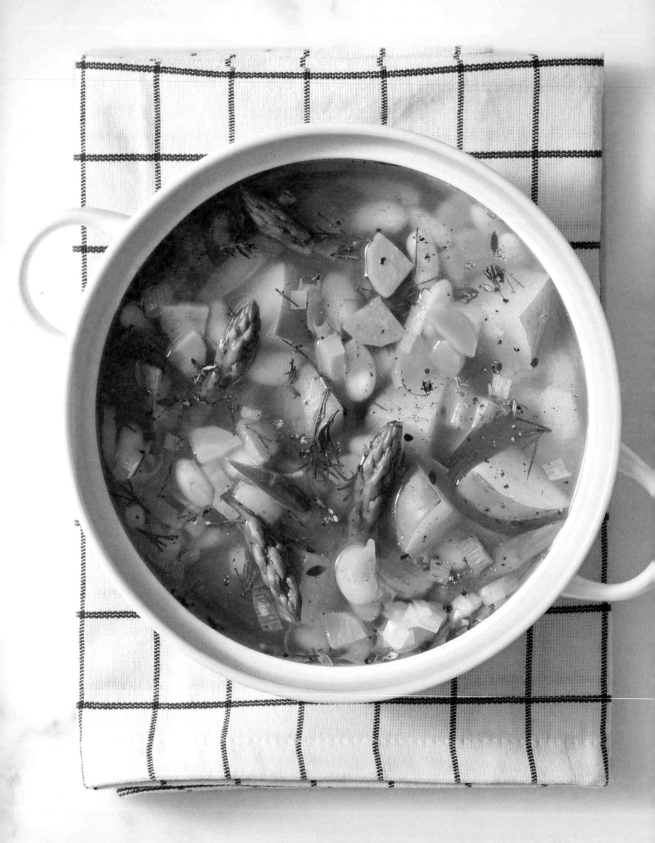

Spring Minestrone

This colorful spring soup—full of healthy veggies like carrots, leeks, and asparagus—can be prepped in a mere 20 minutes.

PREP: 20 MINUTES   TOTAL: 50 MINUTES

2 tablespoons olive oil

2 medium carrots, peeled and chopped

1 medium leek, thinly sliced

8 sprigs fresh thyme, tied together

Salt

3 large red potatoes, chopped

2 quarts low-sodium vegetable or chicken broth

1 bunch asparagus, trimmed and sliced

1 (15-ounce) can navy beans, rinsed and drained (optional)

2 tablespoons chopped fresh dill

Ground black pepper

1. In an 8-quart saucepot, heat the olive oil on medium. Add the carrots, leek, thyme, and ¼ teaspoon salt. Cook 8 minutes, stirring. Add the potatoes and broth. Partially cover the pot and heat to boiling on high; reduce the heat to a simmer. Cook until the potatoes are tender, about 25 minutes.

2. Add the asparagus and simmer until tender, about 3 minutes. Discard the thyme. Stir in the navy beans (if using), dill, ¼ teaspoon salt, and ½ teaspoon pepper.

SERVES 4: About 330 calories, 7g protein, 62g carbohydrates, 7g fat (1g saturated), 7g fiber, 1,030mg sodium.

TIP

When you're trimming and slicing the asparagus, leave the stalks rubber-banded together. Snap off the ends and cut through the rest of the stalks with a few quick strokes to slice all the asparagus in seconds.

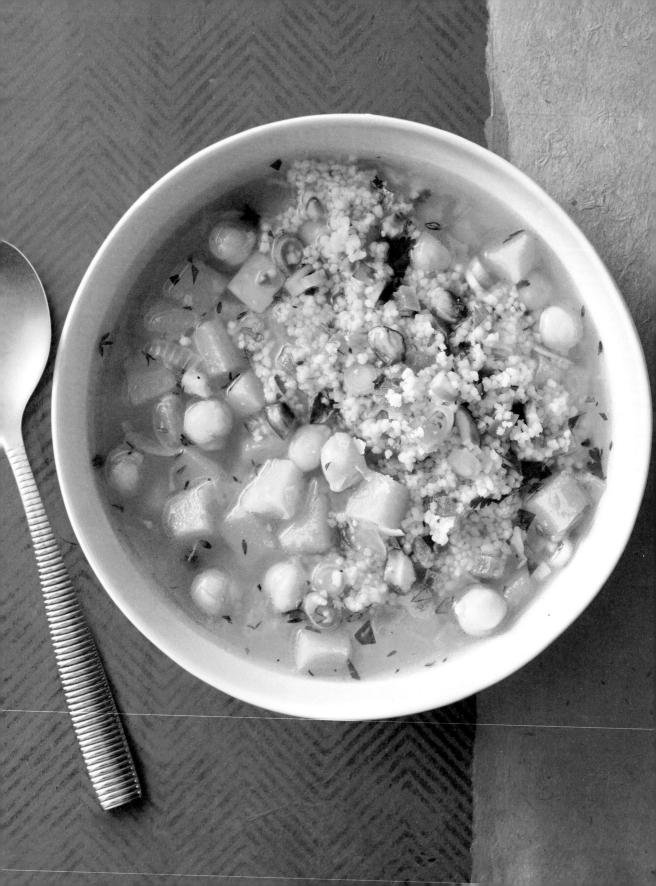

Butternut Squash & White Bean Soup

Cozy up on a chilly fall night with this sweet squash soup.

PREP: **20 MINUTES**   TOTAL: **45 MINUTES**

1 large butternut squash

2 tablespoons olive oil

1 onion, chopped

2 cloves garlic, finely chopped

1 (1-inch) piece peeled fresh ginger, finely chopped

6 cups low-sodium chicken broth

6 sprigs fresh thyme

1 (15-ounce) can white beans, rinsed and drained

1 (15-ounce) can chickpeas, rinsed and drained

½ cup whole-grain couscous

¼ cup roasted pistachios, finely chopped

¼ cup dried apricots, finely chopped

¼ cup fresh cilantro, chopped

1 green onion, sliced

1. Cut the neck from the butternut squash (reserve the base for another use). Peel and cut the neck into ½-inch pieces. Heat 1 tablespoon of the olive oil in a nonstick skillet on medium. Add the squash and cook, covered and stirring occasionally, for 8 minutes.

2. Meanwhile, heat the remaining olive oil in a Dutch oven on medium. Add the onion and cook, covered and stirring occasionally, for 6 minutes. Stir in the garlic and ginger and cook 1 minute.

3. Add the broth, thyme, and butternut squash and bring to a boil. Using a fork, mash the white beans and add them to the soup along with the chickpeas.

4. Cook the couscous as the label directs; fluff it with a fork and fold in the pistachios, apricots, cilantro, and green onion. Serve the soup topped with the couscous mixture.

SERVES 4: About 560 calories, 26g protein, 88g carbohydrates, 16g fat (2g saturated), 19g fiber, 385mg sodium.

Cauliflower Soup

Short on time? This quick and easy soup will warm
you up while filling your body with veggies.

CHIVE OIL

1 bunch fresh chives

½ cup canola or grapeseed oil

SOUP

2 tablespoons extra-virgin olive oil

1 medium onion, chopped

1 leek, chopped

Salt

2 cloves garlic, finely chopped

**1 small head cauliflower (about 2 pounds),
   cored and sliced**

4 cups low-sodium chicken broth

½ cup heavy cream

Cracked black pepper, for serving (optional)

1. Make the chive oil: In a blender, puree
the chives and oil until smooth. Transfer to a
small saucepan and cook on medium until
the mixture begins to simmer, about 3 minutes.
Pour through a coffee filter set over a
measuring cup. Set aside.

2. Heat the olive oil in a large pot on medium.
Add the onion, leek, and ½ teaspoon salt and
cook, covered, stirring occasionally, until very
tender but not browned, 10 to 12 minutes.

3. Stir in the garlic and cook 1 minute. Add the
cauliflower, broth, and cream and simmer until
the cauliflower is tender, 15 to 18 minutes.

4. Using a handheld immersion blender, puree
until smooth. (You can also use a standard
blender and puree the mixture in batches.)

5. Serve the soup drizzled with chive oil and
cracked pepper, if desired.

SERVES 4: About 245 calories, 8g protein,
14g carbohydrates, 19g fat (10g saturated),
3g fiber, 355mg sodium.

TIP

For a quicker alternative, ditch the fresh
cauliflower and replace it with a package
of frozen cauliflower and 1 small coarsely
grated russet potato.

Lemon-Dill Chicken Meatball Soup

This light and satisfying supper is exceptionally good,
and it's good for you!

PREP: **20 MINUTES**   TOTAL: **35 MINUTES**

2 tablespoons olive oil

2 carrots, sliced

2 stalks celery, sliced

1 small onion, chopped

5 cups lower-sodium chicken broth

3 cups water

1¾ cups bulgur

12 ounces ground chicken breast

¼ cup finely chopped fresh dill

1 teaspoon grated lemon zest

Salt

¼ teaspoon ground black pepper

1. Heat the oil in a 6- to 7-quart saucepot over medium heat. Add the carrots, celery, and onion; cook 10 minutes, stirring occasionally.

2. Add the broth and water; heat to boiling over high. Stir in the bulgur. Reduce the heat; simmer 8 to 10 minutes, or until the bulgur is almost tender.

3. Meanwhile, combine the ground chicken, dill, lemon zest, ¼ teaspoon salt, and the pepper. Form the chicken mixture into 1-inch balls; add to the simmering soup along with ¼ teaspoon salt. Cook 6 minutes, or until the meatballs are cooked through.

SERVES 4: About 435 calories, 22g protein, 53g carbohydrates, 16g fat (1g saturated), 9g fiber, 925mg sodium.

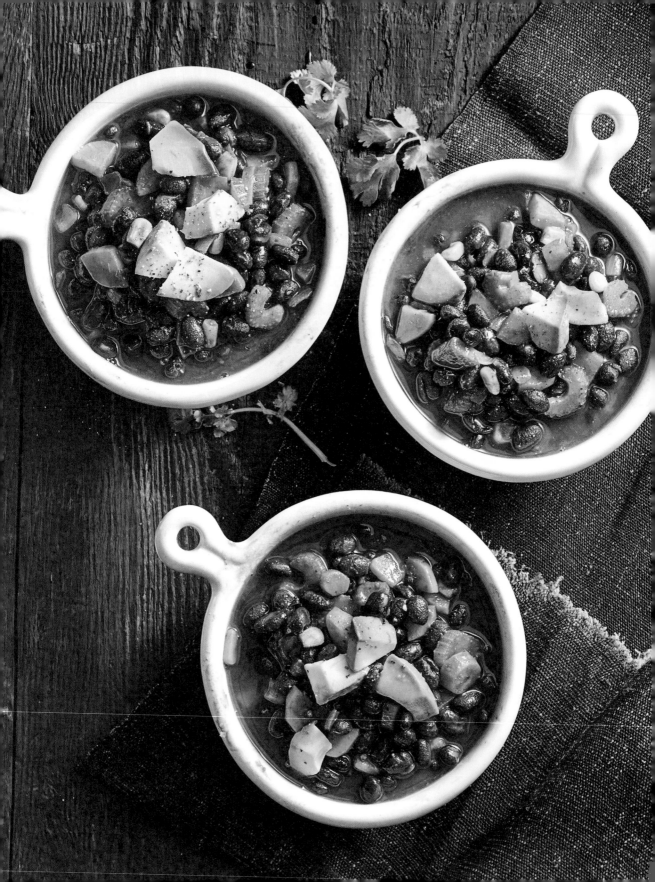

Smoky Vegan Black Bean Soup

Vegetables are the true star of this hearty, healthy soup recipe, making it a perfect option for a meatless Monday meal.

PREP: 20 MINUTES   TOTAL: 4 HOURS 30 MINUTES

2 tablespoons extra-virgin olive oil

2 medium carrots, peeled and chopped

2 stalks celery, sliced

1 medium onion, finely chopped

¼ cup tomato paste

3 cloves garlic, crushed with a garlic press

1½ teaspoons ground cumin

3 cups low-sodium vegetable or chicken broth

3 (15-ounce) cans low-sodium black beans, undrained

1 cup frozen corn

Avocado chunks and cilantro leaves, for serving

1. In a 12-inch skillet, heat the olive oil on medium-high. Add the carrots, celery, and onion. Cook until starting to brown, stirring occasionally, 6 to 8 minutes. Add the tomato paste, garlic, and cumin. Cook, stirring, until the garlic is golden and the tomato paste has browned, 1 to 2 minutes. Stir in ½ cup broth, scraping up any browned bits on the bottom of the skillet.

2. Transfer the contents of the skillet to a 6– to 8-quart slow-cooker bowl, along with the beans, corn, and remaining broth. Cover and cook on High for 4 hours or on Low for 6 hours. Serve with avocado and cilantro.

SERVES 6: About 325 calories, 14g protein, 51g carbohydrates, 11g fat (1g saturated), 19g fiber, 535mg sodium.

Winter Squash & Lentil Stew

This soup recipe warms chilly fingers and toes with seasonal flavors of sweet butternut squash and savory lentils. Seconds, anyone? See photo on page 11.

PREP: 15 MINUTES   **TOTAL:** 35 MINUTES

2 medium shallots, thinly sliced

1 tablespoon peeled fresh ginger, finely chopped

1 tablespoon vegetable oil

1 teaspoon ground coriander

½ teaspoon ground cardamom

1 small butternut squash, peeled, seeded, and cut into 1½-inch chunks

1 pound green lentils, picked over

6 cups low-sodium chicken or vegetable broth

Salt

5 cups packed baby spinach

1 tablespoon cider vinegar

Ground black pepper

1. In a pressure-cooker pot on medium, cook the shallots and ginger in the oil until the shallots are golden, stirring occasionally, about 5 minutes. Add the coriander and cardamom; cook 1 minute, stirring. Add the squash, lentils, broth, and ¼ teaspoon salt.

2. Cover, lock, and bring up to pressure on high. Reduce the heat to medium-low. Cook 12 minutes. Release the pressure by using the quick-release function.

3. Stir in the spinach, vinegar, and ½ teaspoon each salt and pepper.

SERVES 6: About 325 calories, 19g protein, 57g carbohydrates, 4g fat (1g saturated), 15g fiber, 705mg sodium.

Mixed Greens & Herb Toss Salad

Sprinkle in some edible flowers for a touch of spring.

TOTAL: **10 MINUTES**

6 cups mixed spring greens (like Bibb, pea shoots, and mâche), torn

2 cups mixed herbs (like tarragon, dill, mint, and chives), chopped

1 cup shelled edamame

¼ cup extra-virgin olive oil

1 tablespoon fresh lemon juice

2 teaspoons Dijon mustard

1 teaspoon honey

Kosher salt and ground black pepper

1 small shallot, finely chopped

Soft-cooked eggs and edible flowers, for serving (optional)

1. In a large bowl, toss the greens and herbs. Fold in the edamame.

2. In a small bowl, whisk together the oil, lemon juice, mustard, honey, and ¼ teaspoon each salt and pepper; stir in the shallot.

3. Gently toss the salad with the dressing and top with eggs and flowers, if desired.

SERVES 6: About 125 calories, 3g protein, 6g carbohydrates, 10g fat (1g saturated), 2g fiber, 180mg sodium.

TIP

Edible flowers can be found at specialty grocery stores or ordered online.

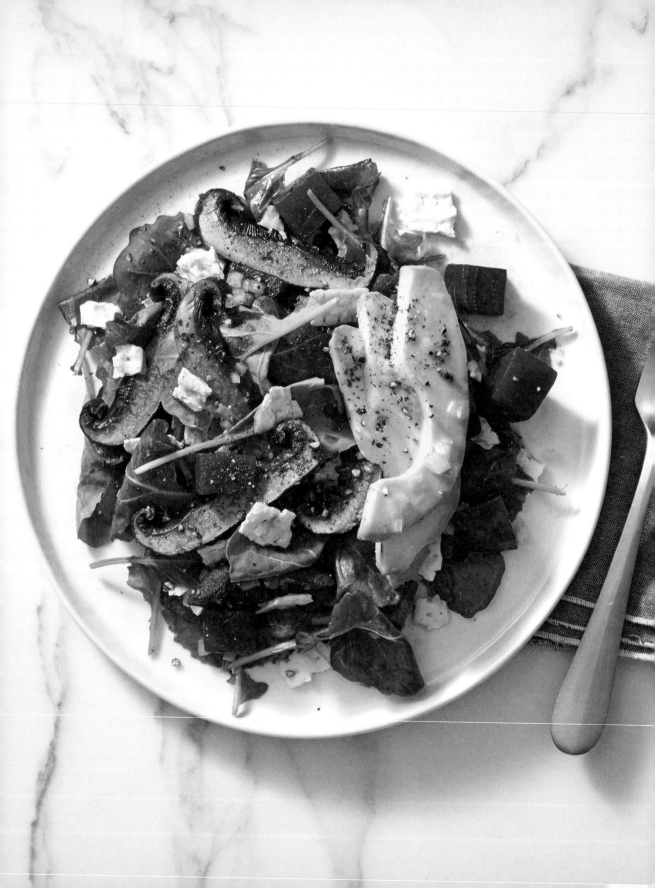

Beet, Mushroom & Avocado Salad

This heart-healthy salad is loaded with antioxidants, fiber-filled vegetables, and healthy unsaturated fats (hello, avocado!).

PREP: 10 MINUTES   **TOTAL: 30 MINUTES**

4 medium portobello mushroom caps

Nonstick cooking spray

Salt

¼ cup fresh lemon juice

3 tablespoons extra-virgin olive oil

1 small shallot, finely chopped

Ground black pepper

5 ounces baby kale

8 ounces precooked beets, chopped

2 ripe avocados, thinly sliced

2 sheets whole wheat matzo, crushed into bite-size pieces

1. Preheat the oven to 450°F.

2. On a large rimmed baking sheet, spray the portobello mushroom caps with nonstick cooking spray and sprinkle with ½ teaspoon salt; roast until tender, about 20 minutes. Let cool, then thinly slice them.

3. In a bowl, whisk together the lemon juice, oil, shallot, and ¼ teaspoon each salt and pepper; toss half the dressing with the baby kale and beets. Divide the mixture among four serving plates and top with the avocado slices, matzo, and sliced portobellos. Serve the remaining dressing on the side.

SERVES 4: About 370 calories, 7g protein, 32g carbohydrates, 26g fat (4g saturated), 11g fiber, 490mg sodium.

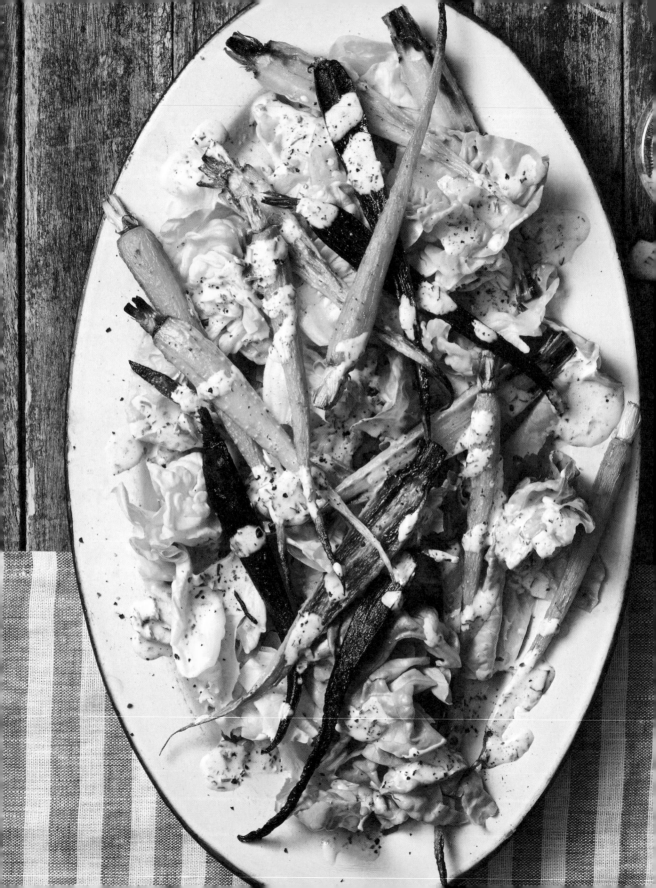

Green Goddess Carrot Salad

With a light buttermilk dressing, this colorful carrot salad is the perfect start to any summer meal.

1 pound slim baby carrots, trimmed and cut lengthwise in half (or in quarters if large)

1 tablespoon olive oil

Salt

¾ cup buttermilk

½ cup mayonnaise

⅓ cup plain Greek yogurt

4 anchovies or 2 teaspoons anchovy paste

2 tablespoons fresh lemon juice

1 tablespoon Dijon mustard

1 small clove garlic

Pinch of sugar

Ground black pepper

½ cup loosely packed fresh parsley

¼ cup packed fresh basil

3 tablespoons fresh tarragon

2 tablespoons snipped fresh chives

1 head Bibb lettuce, leaves separated and torn

1. Preheat the oven to 425°F. On a large rimmed baking sheet, toss the carrots with the oil and ½ teaspoon salt. Roast until the carrots are crisp-tender and the edges are slightly caramelized, 20 to 25 minutes; cool completely.

2. Meanwhile, prepare the green goddess dressing: In a blender, puree the buttermilk, mayonnaise, Greek yogurt, anchovies, lemon juice, mustard, garlic, sugar, ¾ teaspoon salt, and ¼ teaspoon pepper until smooth. Add the parsley, basil, tarragon, and chives; pulse until the herbs are finely chopped. The dressing can be refrigerated up to 1 week. Makes about 2 cups.

3. To serve, arrange the carrots over the lettuce leaves. Drizzle with 1 cup of the dressing.

SERVES 4: About 200 calories, 4g protein, 13g carbohydrates, 15g fat (3g saturated), 4g fiber, 775mg sodium.

Radicchio Salad with Roasted Fennel & Shrimp

Serve this flavorful, protein-packed salad on a thick slice of toast for a hearty meal. See photo on page 6.

PREP: 20 MINUTES   TOTAL: 30 MINUTES

1 bulb fennel, sliced

1 red onion, sliced

1 tablespoon olive oil

Kosher salt and ground black pepper

6 slices bacon

¾ pound peeled and deveined medium (26- to 30-count) shrimp

2 tablespoons balsamic vinegar

1½ tablespoons fresh lemon juice

1 teaspoon sugar

1 medium head radicchio (about 8 ounces), halved, cored, and thinly sliced

1 cup fresh flat-leaf parsley leaves

4 thick slices whole-grain sourdough bread, toasted

Shaved Manchego cheese, for serving (optional)

1. Preheat the oven to 450°F.

2. On a large rimmed baking sheet, toss the fennel and onion with the oil, ¼ teaspoon salt, and ¼ teaspoon pepper. Roast until tender, 10 to 12 minutes.

3. Meanwhile, cook the bacon in a large skillet until crisp and then transfer it to a paper towel–lined plate to drain; discard all but 1 tablespoon of the bacon drippings. Let the bacon cool for a few minutes, then break it into pieces.

4. Season the shrimp with ¼ teaspoon salt and ¼ teaspoon pepper. Add the shrimp to the bacon fat in the skillet and cook on medium-high heat until opaque throughout, 2 to 3 minutes per side.

5. In a large bowl, whisk together the balsamic vinegar, lemon juice, sugar, ¼ teaspoon salt, and ¼ teaspoon pepper. Toss the dressing with the sliced radicchio, roasted vegetables, cooked bacon, sautéed shrimp, and parsley.

6. Serve the salad over the toasts and top with shaved Manchego cheese, if desired.

SERVES 4: About 440 calories, 24g protein, 41g carbohydrates, 21g fat (5g saturated), 5g fiber, 1,295mg sodium.

TIP

If you omit the bacon, you'll drop 75 calories, 6g fat, 2g saturated fat, and 210mg sodium.

Feta-Dill Greek Caesar

This grilled twist on a classic is perfect for summer barbecues. See photo on page 32.

See photo on page 32.

PREP: **10 MINUTES**   TOTAL: **15 MINUTES**

4 ounces feta cheese

⅔ cup extra-virgin olive oil

⅓ cup plain nonfat Greek yogurt

3 tablespoons fresh lemon juice

1 clove garlic

Salt and ground black pepper

¼ cup packed fresh dill, chopped

3 romaine lettuce hearts

¼ cup roasted sunflower seeds

1. Preheat the grill to medium.

2. In a blender or food processor, puree the feta, oil, yogurt, lemon juice, garlic, and salt and pepper to taste. Transfer to a medium bowl; stir in the dill.

3. Cut the romaine hearts in half lengthwise; grill until charred in spots, about 2 minutes per side. Serve immediately, drizzled with yogurt dressing and sprinkled with sunflower seeds.

SERVES 6: About 325 calories, 6g protein, 5g carbohydrates, 32g fat (7g saturated), 1g fiber, 265mg sodium.

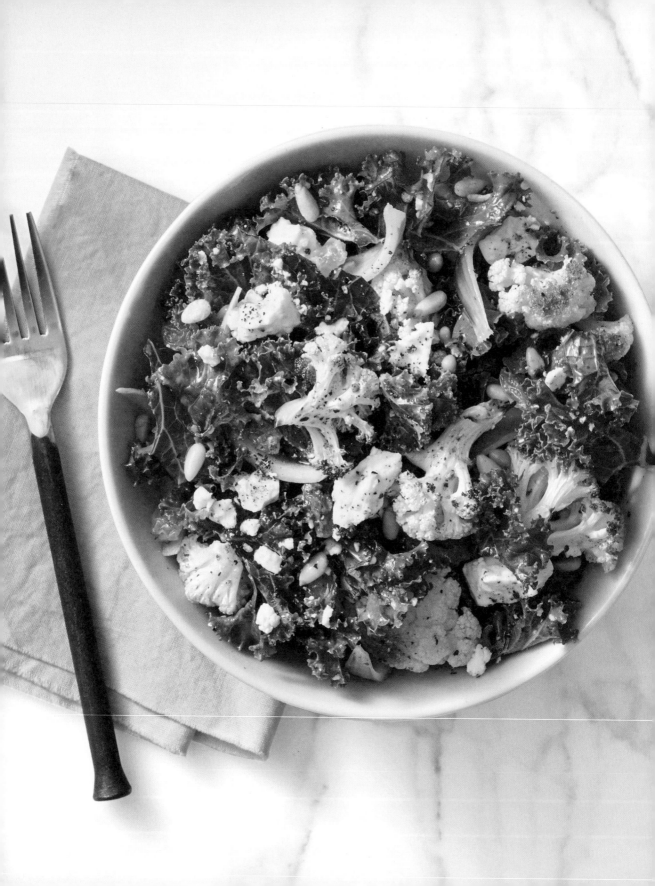

Kale & Roasted Cauliflower Salad

Roasted cauliflower and fresh kale come together in a salad recipe designed to keep your heart healthy and your belly full.

PREP: 10 MINUTES   TOTAL: 35 MINUTES

1 pound cauliflower florets

5 tablespoons extra-virgin olive oil

Salt and ground black pepper

¼ cup fresh lemon juice

1 bunch kale, ribs removed and leaves chopped

¼ small red onion, very thinly sliced

⅓ cup crumbled feta cheese

⅓ cup golden raisins

⅓ cup pine nuts, toasted

1. Preheat the oven to 450°F.

2. On a large rimmed baking sheet, toss the cauliflower florets with 2 tablespoons of the oil and ⅛ teaspoon each salt and pepper. Roast until the stems are tender, about 25 minutes.

3. In a large bowl, whisk the lemon juice, the remaining 3 tablespoons oil, and ½ teaspoon salt. In a large bowl, toss the kale with the dressing. Let stand at least 5 minutes.

4. To the kale, add the roasted cauliflower, onion, feta, golden raisins, and pine nuts. Toss until well combined, and serve.

SERVES 4: About 370 calories, 10g protein, 27g carbohydrates, 28g fat (5g saturated), 6g fiber, 475mg sodium.

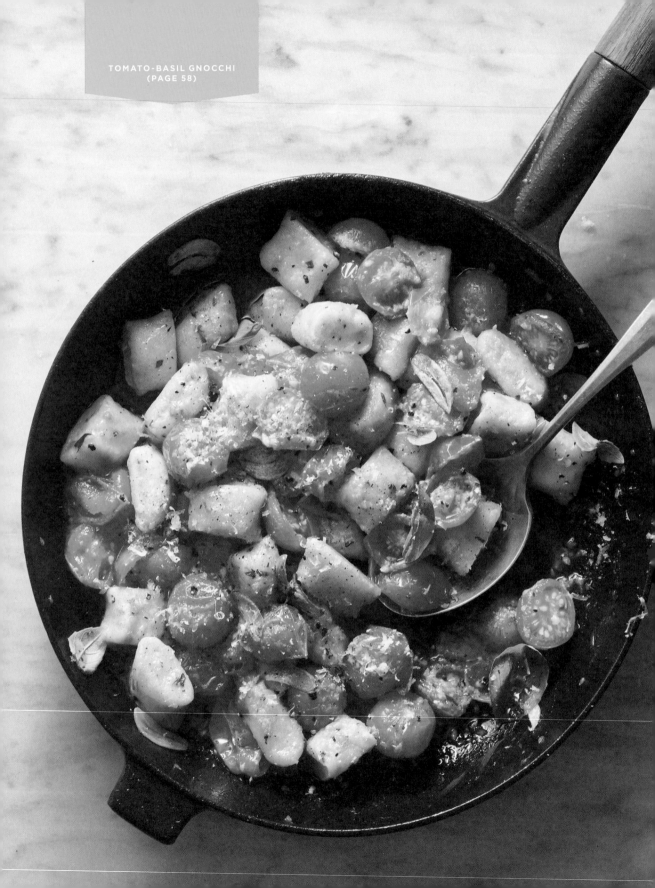

TOMATO-BASIL GNOCCHI
(PAGE 58)

3 | Grains, Beans & Potatoes

Whole grains are an important part of the Mediterranean diet and are essential to long-lasting energy. Pasta, potato, and quinoa are the stars of the dishes in this chapter, which includes everything from regional fare to classic courses. Many of these recipes also feature heart-healthy modifications, such as spiralized zucchini noodles (or "zoodles") that allow you to feast on your favorites guilt-free. Also, consider swapping traditional pasta for bean-based alternatives. They offer the same delicious texture with added protein and oomph!

Pea Pesto Pappardelle · · · · · · · · · · · · · · · 55

Creamy Spaghetti & Zoodles · · · · · · · · · 57

Tomato-Basil Gnocchi · · · · · · · · · · · · · · · 58

Linguine with Tuna & Chiles · · · · · · · · · 59

Creamy Lemon Chicken Pasta · · · · · · · 61

Spring Veggie &
Goat Cheese Spaghetti · · · · · · · · · · · · · · 63

Penne with Roasted
Tomatoes & Spring Onion Pesto · · · · · 65

Creamy Basil Potato Salad · · · · · · · · · · 66

Spanish Potato Omelet · · · · · · · · · · · · · · 67

Spinach & Gruyère
Potato Casserole · 69

Crispy Smashed Potatoes
with Caper Gremolata · · · · · · · · · · · · · · · 70

Cherry Tomato Casserole
with White Beans & Basil · · · · · · · · · · · · 71

Tahini-Lemon Quinoa with
Asparagus Ribbons · · · · · · · · · · · · · · · · · · 73

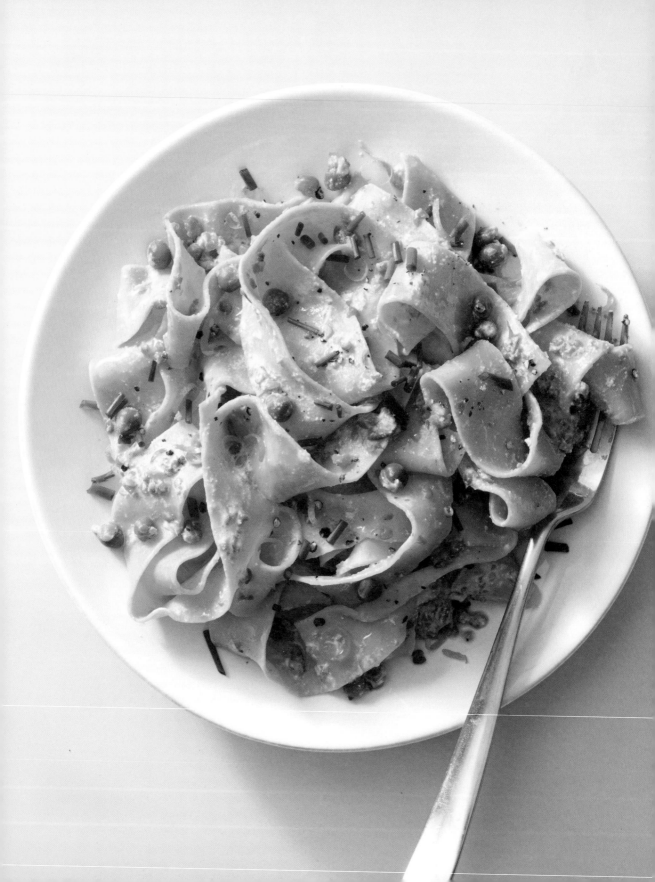

Pea Pesto Pappardelle

This five-ingredient pasta is basically spring on a plate.

PREP: 5 MINUTES   TOTAL: 25 MINUTES

12 ounces whole-grain pappardelle

1½ cups fresh or frozen (thawed) peas

½ cup ricotta cheese

1 teaspoon lemon zest

Salt and ground black pepper

Chopped fresh chives,
   for serving (optional)

1. Cook the pappardelle as the label directs. Reserve ½ cup of the cooking water; drain and then return the pasta to the pot and keep warm.

2. While the pasta is cooking, pulse 1 cup of the peas in the food processor until roughly chopped. Add the ricotta and lemon zest and pulse a few times to combine; there should still be some pieces of chopped peas. Season with salt and pepper to taste.

3. Add the ricotta mixture, the remaining ½ cup peas, and the reserved pasta water to the pasta in the pot; toss to combine. Sprinkle with chopped chives, if desired.

SERVES 4: About 430 calories, 19g protein, 70g carbohydrates, 7g fat (3g saturated), 5g fiber, 100mg sodium.

TIP

Pastas made with chickpea, lentil, bean, or pea flour can boost mineral content and add a *ton* of extra protein and fiber (up to 20 grams of each depending on brand and type). **Added bonus:** These pastas will fill you up and keep you satisfied longer than traditional pasta.

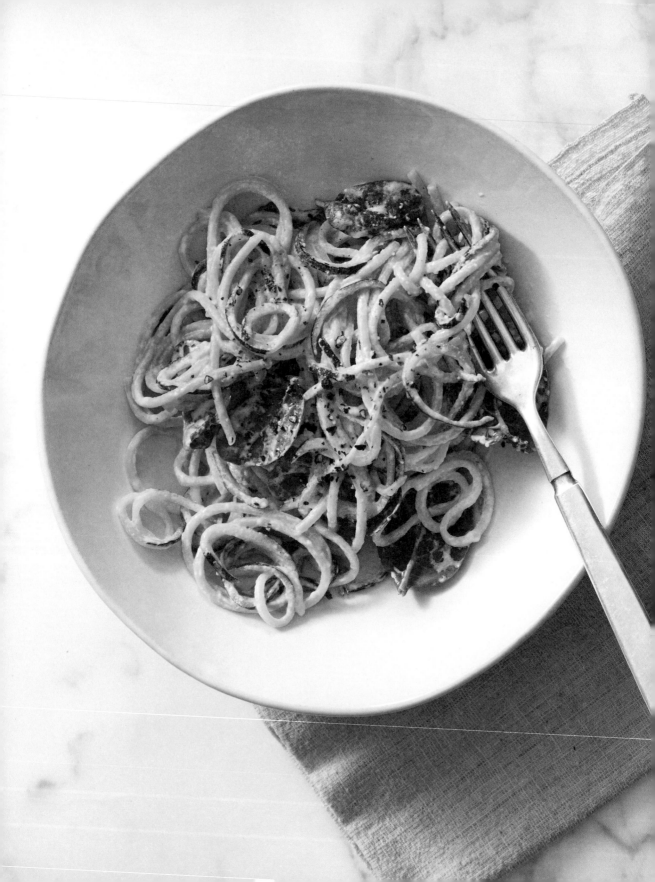

Creamy Spaghetti & Zoodles

Why choose between zucchini noodles and pasta when you can have both?

PREP: 10 MINUTES   TOTAL: 20 MINUTES

8 ounces whole-grain spaghetti

⅓ cup half-and-half

1 clove garlic, smashed

3 sprigs rosemary

⅓ cup freshly grated Parmesan cheese, plus more (optional) for serving

Freshly ground black pepper

2 tablespoons olive oil

1 pound precut zoodles (spiralized zucchini)

Salt

1 teaspoon finely grated lemon zest

5 cups baby spinach

1. Cook the pasta as the label directs, reserving ½ cup of the cooking water before draining.

2. Meanwhile, in a microwave and using a microwave-safe measuring cup, heat the half-and-half with the garlic and rosemary until hot, about 1 minute. Let sit for 5 minutes, then remove and discard the garlic and rosemary. Stir in the Parmesan and ½ teaspoon pepper.

3. During the last 5 minutes of cooking the pasta, heat the olive oil in a large nonstick skillet on medium. Add the zoodles and cook, tossing gently, until just tender, about 2 minutes.

4. Season the zoodles with ¼ teaspoon each salt and pepper and the lemon zest, then fold in the spinach, the cooked and drained pasta, and the cream sauce; add some of the reserved pasta-cooking water if the mixture seems dry. Serve with additional Parmesan, if desired.

SERVES 4: About 345 calories, 13g protein, 49g carbohydrates, 13g fat (3g saturated), 8g fiber, 295mg sodium.

Tomato-Basil Gnocchi

Doughy dumplings made with cheese and herbs?
Now we're talking. See photo on page 52.

PREP: **20 MINUTES**   TOTAL: **45 MINUTES**

GNOCCHI

1 pound fresh ricotta cheese

1 large egg yolk

**1¼ cups white whole-wheat flour,
plus more for rolling**

**2 tablespoons freshly grated
Parmesan cheese, plus more for serving**

½ cup fresh basil, roughly chopped

¼ teaspoon ground nutmeg

Kosher salt and ground black pepper

SAUCE

2 cloves garlic, sliced

3 anchovies

3 tablespoons olive oil

3 cups cherry tomatoes, halved

Salt and ground black pepper

¼ cup fresh basil leaves, torn

Grated Parmesan cheese, for serving

1. Make the gnocchi: In a large bowl, combine the ricotta and egg yolk. Add 1 cup of the flour, the Parmesan, basil, nutmeg, and ¼ teaspoon each salt and pepper. Fold together to make a soft but not sticky dough; do not overmix. Add the remaining ¼ cup flour as needed.

2. Lightly flour a large baking sheet. Divide the ricotta mixture into fourths. Working with lightly floured hands and one portion at a time, roll the gnocchi dough into four 1-inch-wide logs (each about 8 inches long); transfer to the prepared baking sheet and refrigerate, covered loosely with plastic wrap, for 30 minutes.

3. Meanwhile, make the sauce: Heat a large skillet on medium-low and sauté the garlic and anchovies in the oil until the anchovies start to dissolve and the garlic starts to turn golden brown, 2 to 3 minutes. Stir in the tomatoes and cook until they just start to break down, 3 to 4 minutes. Remove from the heat and stir in a pinch of salt, ¼ teaspoon pepper, and the torn basil.

4. Remove the gnocchi logs from the refrigerator and cut them into 1-inch pieces. Bring a large pot of water to a boil; add 1 tablespoon kosher salt. Add the gnocchi and cook until all have risen to the surface, 2 to 3 minutes, then cook 1 minute more. Using a large slotted spoon, transfer the gnocchi to the skillet with the tomatoes, gently tossing to coat. Sprinkle with grated Parmesan, if desired.

SERVES 6: About 335 calories, 14g protein, 28g carbohydrates, 19g fat (8g saturated), 2g fiber, 950mg sodium.

Linguine with Tuna & Chiles

Oil-packed tuna provides extra flavor and premium texture, making this quick and easy pasta dish a true weeknight star.

PREP: 10 MINUTES   TOTAL: 25 MINUTES

12 ounces whole-grain linguine

3 tablespoons olive oil

3 cloves garlic, finely chopped

2 small fresh Thai chiles or 1 jalapeño chile, thinly sliced

2 medium zucchini, thinly sliced

8 ounces mixed mushrooms, thinly sliced

½ teaspoon salt

½ teaspoon ground black pepper

1 jar (6 ounces) tuna packed in olive oil, drained

1. Cook the pasta as the label directs, reserving ½ cup pasta-cooking water.

2. In a 10-inch skillet over medium heat, heat the oil. Add the garlic and chiles and cook 2 minutes, stirring. Add the zucchini, mushrooms, salt, and pepper. Cook 5 minutes, stirring. Remove from the heat.

3. In the pasta pot, toss the cooked pasta, the zucchini mixture, and the tuna, adding reserved pasta water as needed.

SERVES 4: About 490 calories, 23g protein, 70g carbohydrates, 14g fat (3g saturated), 4g fiber, 395mg sodium.

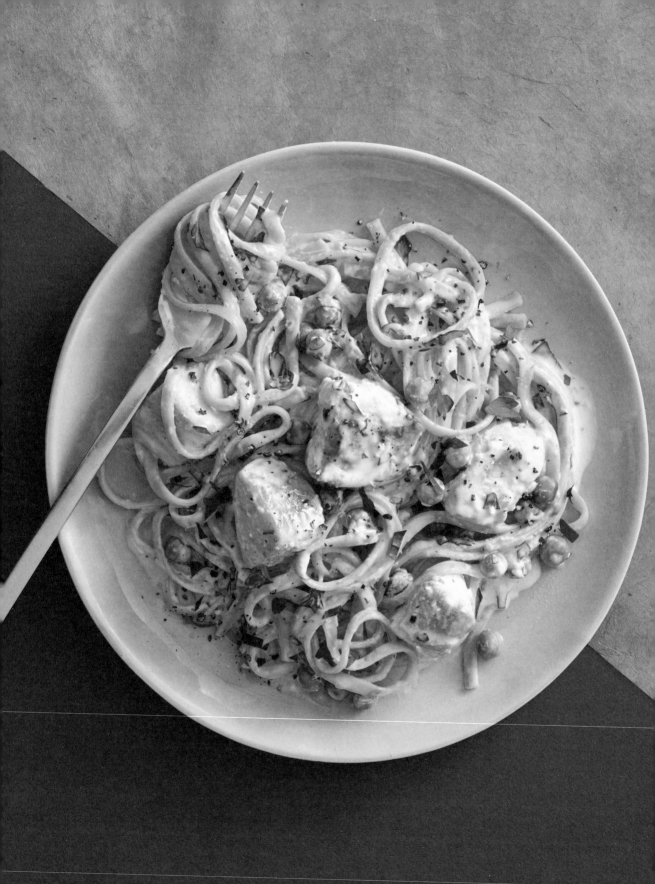

Creamy Lemon Chicken Pasta

Add some tang to your favorite boxed pasta.

12 ounces whole-grain linguine

1 cup frozen (thawed) peas

2 tablespoons olive oil

12 ounces boneless, skinless chicken breasts, cut into 1-inch chunks

Kosher salt and ground black pepper

¼ cup fresh lemon juice

4 ounces low-fat cream cheese, cubed, at room temperature

2 teaspoons finely grated lemon zest

½ cup grated Parmesan cheese

¼ cup flat-leaf parsley, roughly chopped

1. Cook the linguine as the label directs, adding the peas during the last 2 minutes of cooking. Reserve 1 cup of the pasta-cooking water, then drain the pasta and peas and place them in a serving bowl.

2. Meanwhile, heat the oil in a large deep skillet on medium-high. Season the chicken with salt and pepper and cook until golden brown on all sides, 4 to 5 minutes.

3. Add the lemon juice to the skillet and cook, scraping up any browned bits. Add the cream cheese and stir until melted; remove from the heat. Fold in the lemon zest and Parmesan, then the parsley.

4. Toss the mixture from the skillet with the pasta (adding the reserved cooking water, 1 tablespoon at a time, as necessary). Serve immediately.

SERVES 4: About 595 calories, 37g protein, 74g carbohydrates, 18g fat (6g saturated), 3g fiber, 360mg sodium.

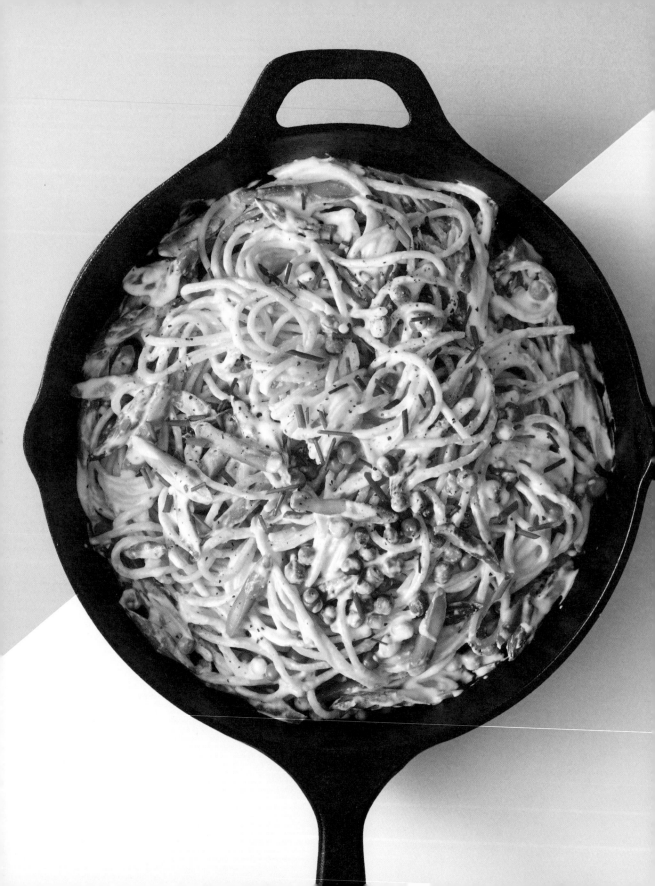

Spring Veggie & Goat Cheese Spaghetti

A classic pasta primavera recipe with fresh spring veggies gets an upgrade thanks to creamy, tangy goat cheese.

PREP: **5 MINUTES**   TOTAL: **20 MINUTES**

2 cups whole milk

1 tablespoon extra-virgin olive oil

12 ounces whole-grain spaghetti or thin linguine

2½ cups water

Salt and ground black pepper

1 pound asparagus, trimmed and sliced on an angle

¼ cup frozen (thawed) peas

4 ounces soft goat cheese, crumbled

3 tablespoons capers, drained

Snipped fresh chives, for garnish

1. In a deep 12-inch skillet, combine the milk, oil, pasta, water, ½ teaspoon salt, and 1 teaspoon pepper. Heat to boiling on high, separating the pasta occasionally with tongs.

2. Add the asparagus and peas. Reduce the heat to maintain a simmer; cook until the pasta is almost al dente and most of the liquid has been absorbed, about 10 minutes, stirring occasionally. Remove the skillet from the heat. Add the goat cheese, capers, and ¼ teaspoon salt, stirring until the cheese has melted. Garnish with chives.

SERVES 4: About 535 calories, 24g protein, 75g carbohydrates, 15g fat (7g saturated), 6g fiber, 715mg sodium.

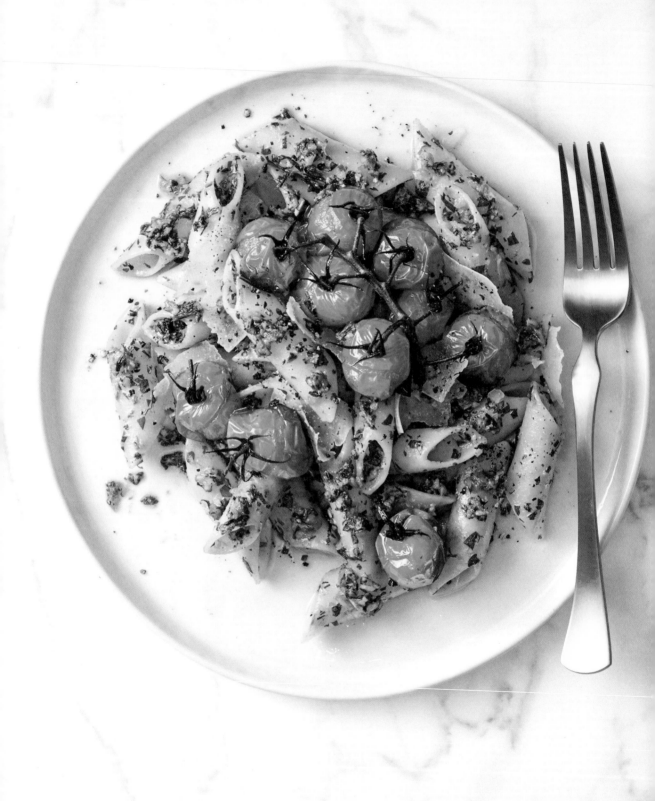

Penne with Roasted Tomatoes & Spring Onion Pesto

Classic pesto meets sweet vine-ripe tomatoes in this delicious dish.

PREP: **5 MINUTES**   TOTAL: **30 MINUTES**

1 pound whole-grain penne pasta

2 medium spring onions, trimmed

1 clove garlic

¼ cup plus 2 teaspoons olive oil

1 pint cherry tomatoes

1 cup parsley

½ cup walnuts

3 tablespoons fresh lemon juice

Salt and ground black pepper

Shaved Pecorino cheese, for serving

1. Preheat the broiler to High. Line a rimmed baking sheet with aluminum foil.

2. Cook the penne as the label directs, reserving ¾ cup of the cooking water; drain the pasta and place it in a serving bowl.

3. Meanwhile, toss the spring onions and garlic with 2 teaspoons of the oil; arrange them in a single layer on the prepared baking sheet and broil until charred, about 4 minutes, turning once.

4. In a heavy 10-inch skillet, heat the remaining ¼ cup oil on medium-high. Add the cherry tomatoes; cover. Cook until they just start to burst, about 5 minutes. Transfer to a plate, reserving the oil in the skillet. Cool the tomatoes slightly.

5. In a food processor, blend the parsley, walnuts, lemon juice, cooked onions and garlic, and the reserved oil until mostly smooth, stopping to stir occasionally. Toss this with the cooked penne, reserved cooking water, and ¾ teaspoon each salt and pepper. To serve, top with shaved Pecorino and the sautéed tomatoes.

SERVES 6: About 475 calories, 16g protein, 61g carbohydrates, 20g fat (4g saturated), 4g fiber, 395mg sodium.

TIP

Spring onions are a more mature version of green onions that feature a small bulb at the base. They are sweeter and mellower than regular onions and the greens have a more intense flavor than green onions. If you do not have spring onions, you can substitute 1 bunch green onions and 1 shallot.

Creamy Basil Potato Salad

Swap tried-and-true mayo for crème fraîche as a tangy substitute.

3 pounds baby red and gold potatoes, scrubbed

Kosher salt

8 ounces crème fraîche, room temperature

1 tablespoon Dijon mustard

2 tablespoons fresh lemon juice

Ground black pepper

3 green onions, thinly sliced, plus more for serving

¾ cup packed fresh basil, thinly sliced, plus more for serving

1. Place the potatoes in a large pot and add enough water to cover by 2 inches. Bring to a boil. Add 1 tablespoon salt, then reduce the heat and gently simmer until tender, 12 to 15 minutes. Drain and run the potatoes under cold water to cool slightly, then spread them out to dry on paper towels. When cool enough to handle, cut the potatoes in half.

2. In a large bowl, whisk together the crème fraîche, mustard, lemon juice, ½ teaspoon salt, and ¼ teaspoon pepper. Add the potatoes, gently tossing to coat, then fold in the green onions and basil.

3. Cover the bowl and let sit 30 minutes or refrigerate up to overnight. Sprinkle with additional green onions and basil before serving.

SERVES 8: About 250 calories, 5g protein, 33g carbohydrates, 12g fat (7g saturated), 3g fiber, 270mg sodium.

Spanish Potato Omelet

Crispy oven-baked potatoes upgrade a basic skillet omelet recipe.

PREP: **10 MINUTES**   TOTAL: **50 MINUTES**

6 large eggs

Salt

1½ pounds Yukon Gold potatoes, peeled and cut into ⅛-inch-thick slices

1¼ cups olive oil

1 large onion, very thinly sliced

Finely chopped parsley, for garnish

1. In a medium bowl, beat the eggs with ¾ teaspoon salt; set aside. In a large bowl, toss the potato slices with ¼ teaspoon salt.

2. In a 10-inch nonstick skillet, heat the oil on medium. Add the potatoes; cook until tender but not falling apart, 10 to 12 minutes, gently turning them occasionally. With a slotted spoon, transfer the potatoes back to the large bowl.

3. To the skillet, add the onion; cook until very tender, about 12 minutes, stirring occasionally. With a slotted spoon, transfer the onion to the large bowl with the potatoes. When the potato-onion mixture has cooled slightly, gently stir in the eggs until well combined.

4. Drain all but 2 teaspoons of the oil from the skillet; heat on medium-high 1 minute. Add the egg-potato mixture to the skillet, spreading it in an even layer; reduce the heat to medium. Cook until the eggs are mostly set and edges are browned, about 7 minutes.

5. Loosen the edges with a rubber spatula. Remove the skillet from the heat and cover it with a large plate; carefully invert the omelet onto the plate, holding the plate and skillet together. Slide the omelet back into skillet with the uncooked side on the bottom. Cook on medium heat until the bottom and center are set, about 3 minutes. Slice and serve warm or at room temperature, garnished with parsley.

SERVES 6: About 245 calories, 8g protein, 22g carbohydrates, 14g fat (3g saturated), 2g fiber, 465mg sodium.

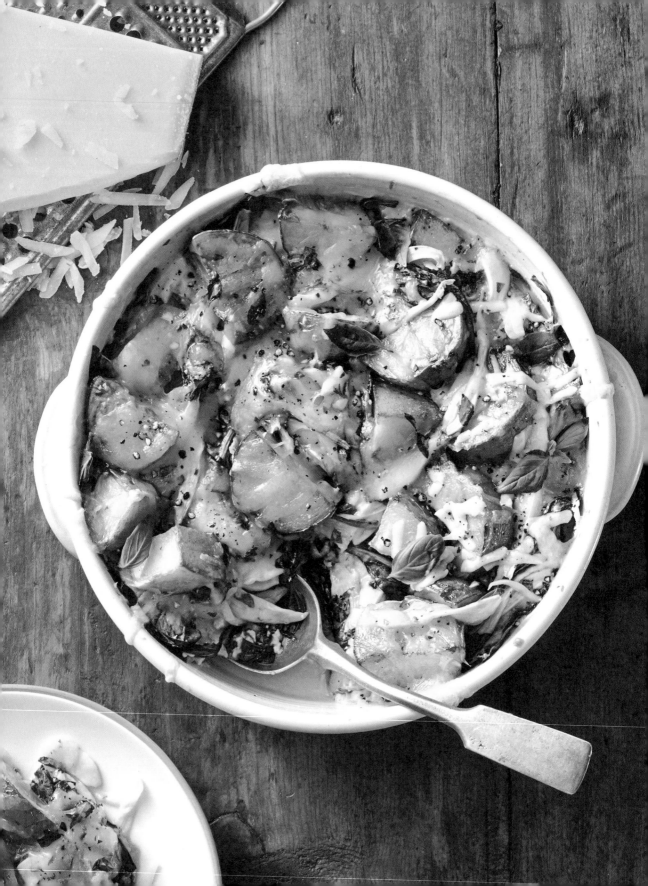

Spinach & Gruyère Potato Casserole

Serve this cheesy bake at your next dinner party and watch your guests swarm.

PREP: 35 MINUTES   **TOTAL: 1 HOUR 15 MINUTES**

1¼ pounds red potatoes, cut into 1-inch chunks

2 tablespoons olive oil

Salt and ground black pepper

4 large eggs

¼ cup half-and-half

2 cups shredded Gruyère cheese

¼ cup chopped fresh basil, plus more (optional) for garnish

¼ cup chopped fresh parsley, plus more (optional) for garnish

3 cloves garlic, finely chopped

3 cups packed fresh spinach, sliced

2 medium bulbs fennel, cored and thinly sliced

1. Preheat the oven to 450°F. In a bowl, toss the potatoes with the oil and ¼ teaspoon each salt and pepper; arrange them in a single layer on a rimmed baking sheet. Roast until golden brown and tender, 20 to 25 minutes. Reduce the oven temperature to 375°F.

2. Meanwhile, whisk together the eggs, half-and-half, and ½ teaspoon salt; stir in the Gruyère, basil, parsley, and garlic. In a large bowl, toss the roasted potatoes, spinach, and fennel with the egg mixture until well combined. Transfer to an oiled 2-quart baking dish; cover with aluminum foil.

3. Bake until the custard has set, 30 to 35 minutes. Uncover and bake another 5 minutes. Garnish with additional basil and parsley, if desired.

SERVES 6: About 305 calories, 16g protein, 23g carbohydrates, 18g fat (7g saturated), 5g fiber, 600mg sodium.

Crispy Smashed Potatoes with Caper Gremolata

A flavor-packed, garlicky parsley rub seeps into the crevices of the potatoes, making this dish irresistible.

PREP: 15 MINUTES   TOTAL: 1 HOUR

2½ pounds new potatoes (about 20)

Kosher salt

4 tablespoons olive oil, plus more for pan

¼ cup sherry vinegar

3 tablespoons capers, drained and chopped

1 tablespoon anchovy paste

1 clove garlic, crushed with a garlic press

¼ cup flat-leaf parsley, finely chopped

1. Place the potatoes in a large pot. Add enough water to cover by 2 inches and bring to a boil. Add 1 tablespoon salt, reduce the heat, and simmer until tender, 18 to 22 minutes. Drain.

2. Meanwhile, arrange one oven rack 6 inches from the broiler and preheat the oven to 450°F. Oil a large rimmed baking sheet. Place each potato on the prepared baking sheet and, using the bottom of a glass, gently press down until the potato is crushed but still intact. Brush the tops with 1 tablespoon of oil and roast 25 minutes.

3. Brush the potatoes with 1 more tablespoon of oil, then broil them until deep golden brown and crisp, 4 to 7 minutes. Sprinkle with ¼ teaspoon salt.

4. While the potatoes cook, in a bowl, combine the vinegar, capers, anchovy paste, garlic, the remaining 2 tablespoons olive oil, and ½ teaspoon salt; stir in the parsley. Drizzle over broiled potatoes and serve immediately.

SERVES 6: About 255 calories, 5g protein, 34g carbohydrates, 11g fat (2g saturated), 3g fiber, 575mg sodium.

Cherry Tomato Casserole with White Beans & Basil

Think of this one-dish wonder like a cheesy,
savory bread pudding.

PREP: **15 MINUTES**   TOTAL: **55 MINUTES**

2 cups (about 5 ounces) hearty whole
wheat bread, cut into 1-inch cubes

2 tablespoons extra-virgin olive oil

2 pounds cherry tomatoes, halved

2 (15-ounce) cans no-salt-added
cannellini beans, rinsed and drained

¼ cup packed fresh basil, chopped

3 cloves garlic, chopped

½ teaspoon crushed red pepper

Kosher salt and ground black pepper

¼ cup grated Parmesan cheese

1. Preheat the oven to 350°F. On a large rimmed baking sheet, toss the bread cubes with the oil. Bake until golden, 8 to 10 minutes, stirring halfway through.

2. Meanwhile, in a large bowl, combine the tomatoes, beans, basil, garlic, crushed red pepper, 1 teaspoon salt, and ¼ teaspoon pepper. Add the toasted bread; toss to combine.

3. Transfer the mixture to a shallow 6- to 7-cup baking dish. Sprinkle with Parmesan; bake until the top is golden, about 40 minutes. Let cool 10 minutes before serving.

SERVES 4: About 400 calories, 18g protein, 52g carbohydrates, 14g fat (3g saturated), 3g fiber, 820mg sodium.

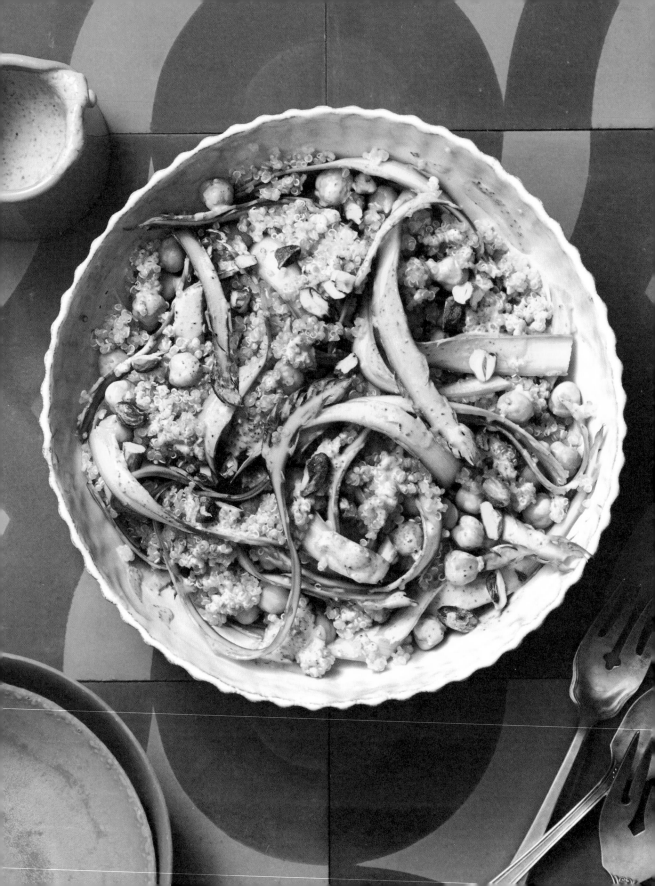

Tahini-Lemon Quinoa with Asparagus Ribbons

We officially declare shaved asparagus ribbons the new zoodles.

PREP: 35 MINUTES   **TOTAL: 2 HOURS 15 MINUTES**

1 (15-ounce) can chickpeas, rinsed and drained

Zest and juice of 1 lemon

Kosher salt and ground black pepper

1 cup quinoa

½ cup tahini

¼ cup fresh lime juice

1 tablespoon honey

1 cup packed fresh mint leaves

½ cup water

1 pound thick asparagus, trimmed

¼ cup shelled pistachios, chopped

1. In a bowl, combine the chickpeas, lemon zest and juice, and a pinch each of salt and pepper. Let sit 20 minutes or refrigerate overnight, then drain.

2. Meanwhile, cook the quinoa as the label directs and season with a pinch of salt.

3. In a blender, puree the tahini, lime juice, honey, mint, water, and ¼ teaspoon salt until smooth, adding additional water if needed; set aside.

4. With a vegetable peeler, shave the asparagus into ribbons, peeling from the woody end up toward the tip. In a bowl, combine the cooked quinoa, asparagus ribbons, and marinated chickpeas. Sprinkle with pistachios, drizzle with tahini dressing, and serve.

SERVES 4: About 525 calories, 20g protein, 64g carbohydrates, 24g fat (3g saturated), 13g fiber, 315mg sodium.

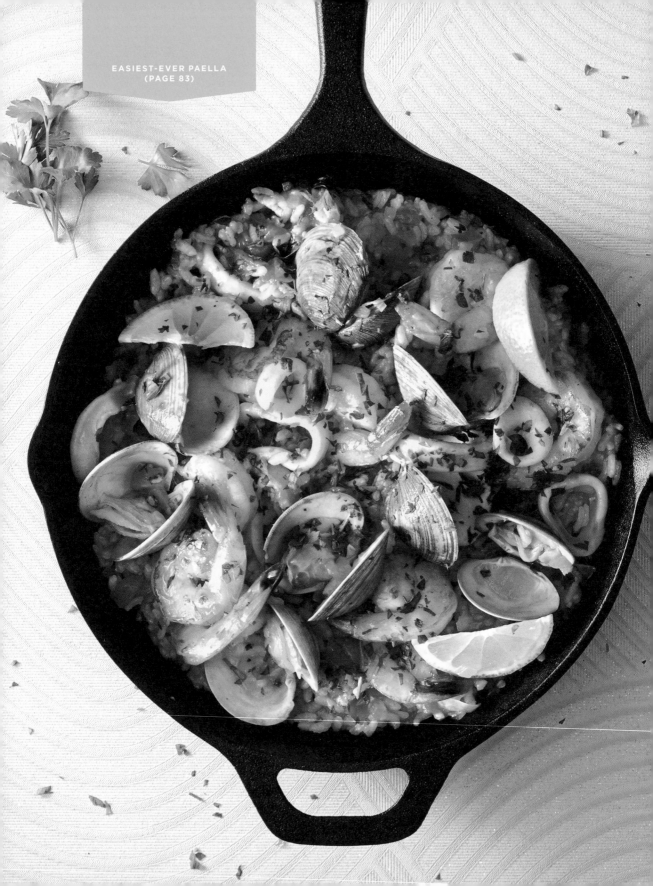

EASIEST-EVER PAELLA
(PAGE 83)

4 | Mains

Lean meats and seafood are your main-dish options on the Mediterranean diet. There's a recipe here for every occasion, from one-pot meals for a lazy night in to dishes that will impress at your next dinner party. A wide variety of spicy, sweet, and savory flavors pair perfectly with proteins in these healthy main dishes. Plus some dishes are rounded out with whole grains or hearty vegetables for a complete meal.

Honey-Ginger Cedar Plank Salmon ·· 77

Honey-Soy-Glazed Salmon
with Peppers 78

Seared Salmon with Lentil Salad ···· 79

Soy-Glazed Cod & Bok Choy 81

Zesty Lemon-Herb Baked Flounder ·· 82

Easiest-Ever Paella 83

Shrimp Packets with Kale Couscous ·· 85

Roasted Cumin Shrimp & Asparagus · 87

Chicken & Red Plum Salad 88

Chipotle Orange Chicken............. 89

Skillet Pesto Chicken & Beans 91

Roasted Baby Vine Tomato
Grilled Chicken 92

Harissa Grilled Chicken Kebabs ···· 93

Sheet Pan Chickpea Chicken......... 95

Chicken Marsala 96

Chicken Souvlaki Skewers........... 97

Lamb Souvlaki with
Cucumber-Mint Salad 99

Moroccan Chicken with
Preserved Lemons & Olives 100

Chicken Cacciatore.................. 101

Skillet Lemon Chicken
with Artichokes 103

Pomegranate-Honey-Glazed
Chicken & Squash 105

Chicken Quinoa Bowls 106

Grilled Lamb & Artichoke Kebabs ··· 107

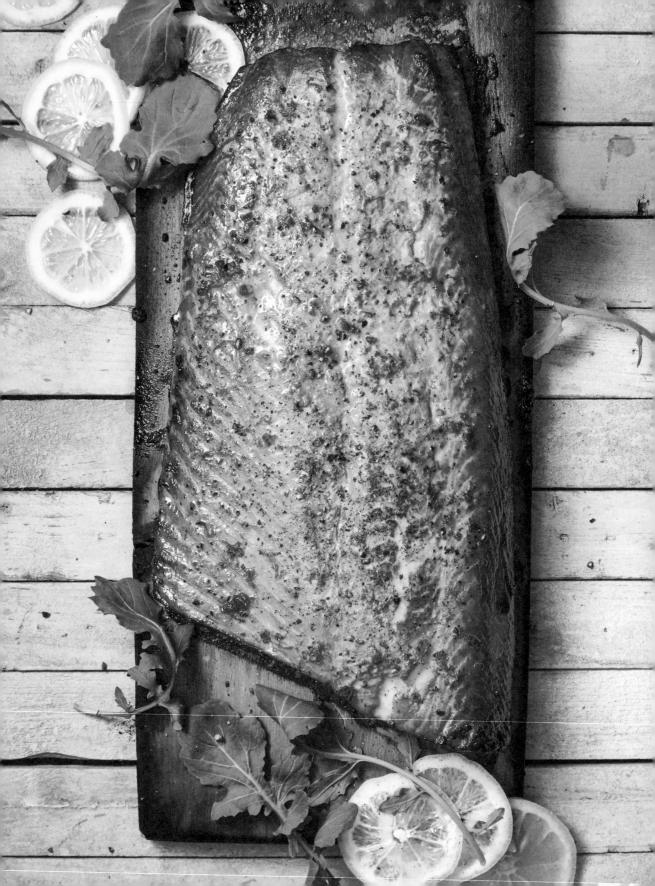

Honey-Ginger Cedar Plank Salmon

This grilled salmon is a total triple threat: sweet, spicy, and earthy.

PREP: **15 MINUTES**   TOTAL: **30 MINUTES**

2 lemons, plus slices for garnish

2 teaspoons grated peeled fresh ginger

Coarsely ground black pepper

1 large piece skin-on wild Alaskan salmon (about 2 pounds)

Salt

3 tablespoons low-sodium soy sauce

2 tablespoons honey

1 tablespoon sriracha sauce

1 clove garlic, crushed with a garlic press

4 cups packed arugula, plus more for garnish

4 miniature seedless cucumbers, thinly sliced

1¼ cups cooked corn kernels (from 2 ears)

½ cup loosely packed fresh cilantro leaves

1. Soak a large cedar grilling plank (about 15 × 7 inches) in water for 1 to 2 hours. When you're ready to cook, preheat the grill to medium.

2. From the lemons, grate 1 teaspoon zest and squeeze ¼ cup juice; set the juice aside. Combine the zest with the ginger and ½ teaspoon pepper; rub this mixture all over the flesh side of the salmon.

3. Place the salmon on the soaked cedar plank, skin side down; sprinkle with ½ teaspoon salt. Grill 20 to 25 minutes, covered, or to desired doneness.

4. Meanwhile, in a medium bowl, whisk together the soy sauce, honey, and sriracha; set aside half. Add the garlic, reserved lemon juice, and ¼ teaspoon salt to the remaining soy sauce mixture; toss with the 4 cups of arugula, cucumbers, corn, and cilantro. Brush the salmon with the reserved soy sauce mixture. Garnish the salmon with arugula and lemon slices and serve with the cucumber-corn salad.

SERVES 8: About 190 calories, 25g protein, 12g carbohydrates, 5g fat (1g saturated), 1g fiber, 530mg sodium.

Honey-Soy-Glazed Salmon with Peppers

This sweet 'n' sticky soy sauce glaze tastes equally delicious on chicken or grilled veggies.

PREP: 5 MINUTES   TOTAL: 25 MINUTES

2 large bell peppers, seeded and thinly sliced

1 medium red onion, thinly sliced

2 tablespoons toasted sesame oil

Salt

3 tablespoons low-sodium soy sauce

2 tablespoons honey

2 teaspoons grated peeled fresh ginger

Ground black pepper

4 (5-ounce) skinless salmon fillets

3 cups cooked brown rice

Fresh basil, for garnish

1. Preheat the oven to 425°F. On a large rimmed baking sheet, toss the bell peppers with the onion, 1 tablespoon of the oil, and ¼ teaspoon salt. Roast until tender, about 20 minutes.

2. In a 2-quart baking dish, whisk together the remaining 1 tablespoon oil, the soy sauce, honey, ginger, and ¼ teaspoon pepper; add the salmon, turning the fillets to coat. Bake until cooked through, 15 to 20 minutes.

3. Serve the salmon with the pepper mixture and the brown rice. Garnish with fresh basil.

SERVES 4: About 505 calories, 36g protein, 51g carbohydrates, 17g fat (3g saturated), 5g fiber, 875mg sodium.

Seared Salmon with Lentil Salad

Keep it lean with this heart-healthy salmon-and-greens dinner.

PREP: **10 MINUTES**   TOTAL: **20 MINUTES**

4 (5-ounce) skinless salmon fillets

Kosher salt and ground black pepper

2 tablespoons plus 2 teaspoons olive oil

2 lemons, halved

2 tablespoons lemon juice

2 teaspoons Dijon mustard

1 teaspoon fresh thyme

½ small red onion, finely chopped

1 (15-ounce) can lentils, rinsed and drained

1 small English (seedless) cucumber, cut into pieces

4 cups baby spinach

¼ cup fresh dill, very roughly chopped

1. Heat a large skillet on medium. Season the salmon fillets with ¼ teaspoon each of salt and pepper. Add 2 teaspoons of the oil to the skillet, then add the salmon and lemon halves, cut sides down, and cook until the salmon is opaque throughout, about 5 minutes per side. Remove the skillet from the heat, let cool, and squeeze the charred lemon halves over the salmon.

2. Meanwhile, in a large bowl, whisk together the lemon juice, mustard, the remaining 2 tablespoons oil, and salt and pepper to taste; stir in the thyme.

3. In a bowl, toss the vinaigrette with the onion and lentils, then fold in the cucumber, spinach, and dill. Serve with the salmon.

SERVES 4: About 350 calories, 37g protein, 19g carbohydrates, 13g fat (2g saturated), 9g fiber, 490mg sodium.

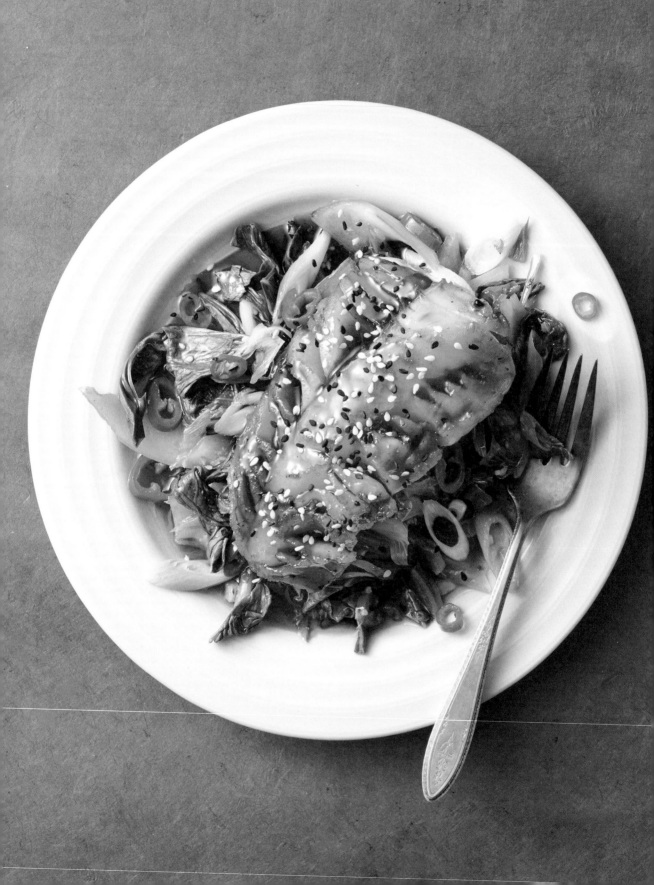

Soy-Glazed Cod & Bok Choy

It only takes sixty seconds in the microwave to
make this sweet glaze come together.

PREP: 10 MINUTES   TOTAL: 30 MINUTES

2 tablespoons honey

2 tablespoons low-sodium soy sauce

1 tablespoon balsamic vinegar

4 (6-ounce) skinless cod fillets

Kosher salt and ground black pepper

1 tablespoon canola oil

3 cloves garlic, finely chopped

4 green onions, thinly sliced

1 small fresh red chile, thinly sliced

1 (1-inch) piece peeled grated ginger

3 large heads bok choy
   (about 2¼ pounds), chopped

Toasted sesame seeds, for serving
   (optional)

1. Position an oven rack 6 inches from the broiler. Preheat the broiler.

2. In a small microwave-safe bowl, whisk together the honey, soy sauce, and balsamic vinegar. Microwave until slightly thickened, 60 to 90 seconds.

3. Pat the cod fillets dry and season with ½ teaspoon salt and ½ teaspoon pepper. Spoon half of the glaze over the cod and brush to evenly coat it. Broil the cod until it is opaque throughout, 6 to 7 minutes, turning if needed. Spoon the remaining glaze over the top.

4. Meanwhile, heat the oil in a large skillet on medium-high. Add the garlic, green onions, chile, and ginger and cook, tossing for 30 seconds. Add the bok choy and ¼ teaspoon salt. Cover and cook for 2 minutes. Uncover and cook, tossing, until the bok choy is tender, 3 to 4 minutes more; add 1 to 2 tablespoons water if necessary. Serve with the glazed cod, sprinkling the fish with sesame seeds, if desired.

SERVES 4: About 265 calories, 31g protein, 17g carbohydrates, 9g fat (1g saturated), 3g fiber, 650mg sodium.

Zesty Lemon-Herb Baked Flounder

These tender flounder fillets, seasoned with lemon slices and crushed croutons, make for a satisfying under-200-calorie meal.

1¼ pounds flounder fillets

Salt and ground black pepper

1 medium lemon, thinly sliced

3 tablespoons olive oil

½ cup whole-grain Italian-seasoned croutons

Chopped fresh parsley, for garnish

1. Preheat the oven to 450°F.

2. In a 3-quart baking dish, arrange the flounder fillets in a single layer; season with ¼ teaspoon each salt and pepper. Top with lemon slices and drizzle with the oil. Bake until the fish just turns opaque in the center, 12 to 15 minutes.

3. Meanwhile, pulse the croutons in a food processor until coarsely crushed. Sprinkle them over the baked flounder. Garnish with chopped parsley.

SERVES 4: About 190 calories, 16g protein, 5g carbohydrates, 12g fat (6g saturated), 0g fiber, 605mg sodium.

TIP

Serve this dish with sautéed greens, like spinach, and whole-grain dinner rolls, if desired.

Easiest-Ever Paella

The sea's most delicious treasures—clams, shrimp, and squid—come together over aromatic Arborio rice in this simple recipe. Who says a fancy seafood dinner has to be a challenge? See photo on page 74.

See photo on page 74.

PREP: 15 MINUTES   TOTAL: 1 HOUR 10 MINUTES

⅓ cup extra-virgin olive oil

8 ounces peeled and deveined large (16- to 20-count) shrimp

8 ounces squid bodies, rinsed, patted dry, and sliced

Salt

1 medium onion, finely chopped

1 (14-ounce) can fire-roasted diced tomatoes, drained

3 cloves garlic, chopped

1½ cups Arborio rice

3½ cups seafood broth

1 (8-ounce) bottle clam juice

12 littleneck clams, scrubbed

Parsley and lemon wedges, for garnish

1. In a deep 12-inch cast-iron skillet, heat the oil on medium-high until hot but not smoking. Add the shrimp, squid, and a pinch of salt. Cook until the shrimp start to brown, about 2 minutes, stirring once. With a slotted spoon, transfer the seafood to a medium bowl.

2. Reduce the heat to medium. Add the onion and tomatoes. Cook 8 minutes, stirring often. Add the garlic; cook 2 minutes. Add the rice; cook 2 minutes, stirring.

3. To the skillet, add the broth and clam juice, stirring to distribute the rice evenly in the pan. Heat to boiling on medium-high. Boil, without stirring, 15 minutes.

4. Nestle the parcooked shrimp and squid and the clams on top of the rice. Cover the skillet with a lid or aluminum foil; cook until clams open and the rice is just tender, another 10 to 16 minutes. Remove from the heat. Let stand, covered, 10 minutes before serving. Garnish with parsley and lemons.

SERVES 6: About 390 calories, 21g protein, 45g carbohydrates, 14g fat (2g saturated), 3g fiber, 935mg sodium.

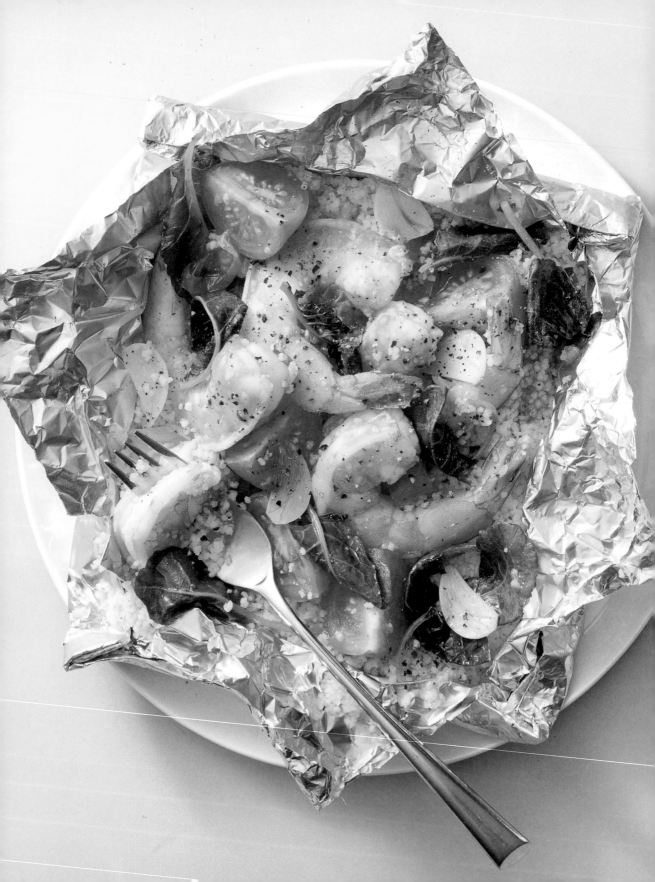

Shrimp Packets with Kale Couscous

Want a stress-free meal? Foil packets are always the answer.

1 cup whole-grain couscous

½ cup water

5 ounces kale

1 pound cocktail tomatoes (like Campari), quartered

2 large cloves garlic, thinly sliced

1 pound peeled and deveined large (16- to 20-count) shrimp

2 tablespoons olive oil

Salt and ground black pepper

1. Preheat the grill to medium-high.

2. In a bowl, combine the couscous and water. Evenly divide the kale among four 12-inch squares of aluminum foil. Top each with one-fourth of the couscous, tomatoes, and garlic. Divide and arrange the shrimp on top, drizzle with oil, and season each packet with ¼ teaspoon each salt and pepper.

3. Cover each packet with another square of foil and fold each edge up and over three times. Transfer to 2 rimmed baking sheets and grill, covered, 15 minutes.

4. Using scissors or a knife, cut an X in the centers. Fold back the triangles to serve.

SERVES 4: About 335 calories, 41g protein, 41g carbohydrates, 9g fat (1g saturated), 5g fiber, 795mg sodium.

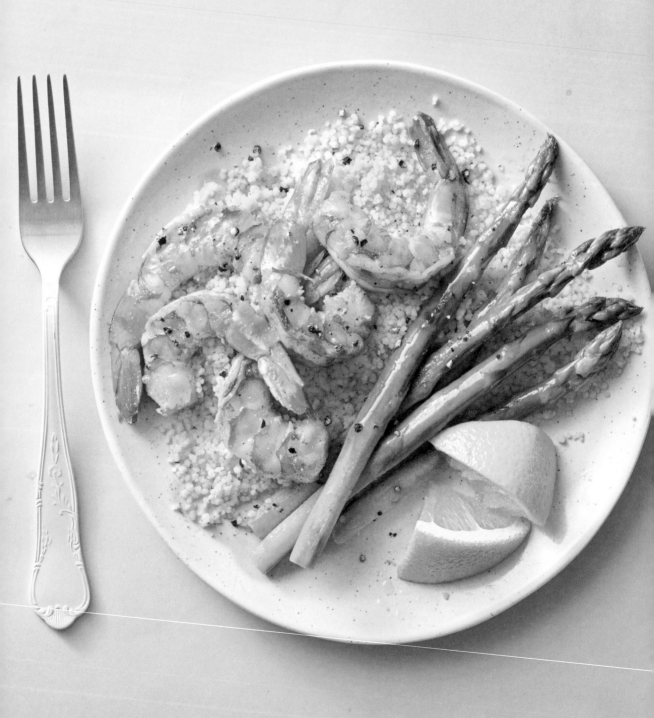

Roasted Cumin Shrimp & Asparagus

Kick up the flavor by adding cumin and cayenne
to this simple shrimp dinner.

PREP: 10 MINUTES   TOTAL: 30 MINUTES

1 cup whole-grain couscous

1 navel orange

1 cup hot water

Kosher salt and ground black pepper

20 (1 pound) peeled and deveined
    large shrimp

½ teaspoon ground cumin

¼ teaspoon cayenne pepper

1 pound thin asparagus, trimmed

2 tablespoons olive oil

1. Place the couscous in a bowl. Add the juice
from half the orange and the hot water; cover
and let sit 15 minutes; fluff with a fork and season
with salt and pepper.

2. Meanwhile, preheat the broiler. Season the
shrimp with the cumin, cayenne pepper, and
salt to taste. Toss the asparagus with the oil
and season with salt and pepper to taste.

3. Place the shrimp and asparagus on a rimmed
baking sheet and broil until the shrimp turn
opaque throughout, about 2 minutes per side,
and the asparagus is just tender.

4. Squeeze the remaining orange half over the
shrimp; serve the shrimp and asparagus with
the couscous.

SERVES 4: About 270 calories, 12g protein,
39g carbohydrates, 8g fat (1g saturated),
4g fiber, 445mg sodium.

Chicken & Red Plum Salad

Charred plums make this nutty salad a summer standout.

PREP: 5 MINUTES   TOTAL: 20 MINUTES

4 (6-ounce) boneless, skinless chicken breasts

2 tablespoons plus 1 teaspoon olive oil

Salt and ground black pepper

4 red plums, cut into 1-inch wedges

2 green onions, thinly sliced

6 cups baby arugula

½ cup fresh dill, very roughly chopped

¼ cup roasted almonds, chopped

1. Preheat the grill to medium. Rub the chicken breasts with 1 teaspoon of the oil and season with salt and pepper. In a large bowl, toss the red plums with 1 tablespoon of the oil and season with salt and pepper.

2. Grill the chicken until cooked through (165°F), 5 to 7 minutes per side. Transfer to a cutting board. Grill the plums until just charred, 2 to 3 minutes per side; return to the large bowl and toss with the remaining 1 tablespoon oil and the green onions.

3. Slice the chicken and add it to the bowl along with any juices; toss to combine. Fold in the baby arugula, fresh dill, and roasted almonds.

SERVES 4: About 355 calories, 38g protein, 12g carbohydrates, 17g fat (3g saturated), 3g fiber, 345mg sodium.

Chipotle Orange Chicken

With its bold and bright citrus flavor, this simple
grilled chicken is a hit. See photo on page 2.

See photo on page 2.

PREP: 5 MINUTES TOTAL: 35 MINUTES

1 tablespoon light brown sugar

2 teaspoons chipotle chile powder

1 teaspoon ground cumin

1 teaspoon garlic powder

½ teaspoon onion powder

Salt and ground black pepper

12 small chicken thighs (about 4 pounds),
trimmed of excess skin

2 tablespoons extra-virgin olive oil

2 small oranges, cut into quarters

2 green onions, thinly sliced

1. Preheat the grill to medium.

2. In a small bowl, combine the brown sugar, chipotle chile powder, cumin, garlic powder, onion powder, and 1 teaspoon each salt and pepper. In a large bowl or a 3-quart baking dish, toss the chicken with the oil; sprinkle the spice mixture on top, then rub the spices into the chicken to coat it evenly.

3. Grill the chicken, covered, until chicken is cooked through (165°F), 20 to 25 minutes, turning once. Grill the oranges until grill marks appear, 5 to 10 minutes. Transfer the chicken to a serving platter. Squeeze the juice from the grilled oranges over the chicken. Garnish with the green onions.

SERVES 6: About 480 calories, 42g protein, 6g carbohydrates, 31g fat (8g saturated), 1g fiber, 535mg sodium.

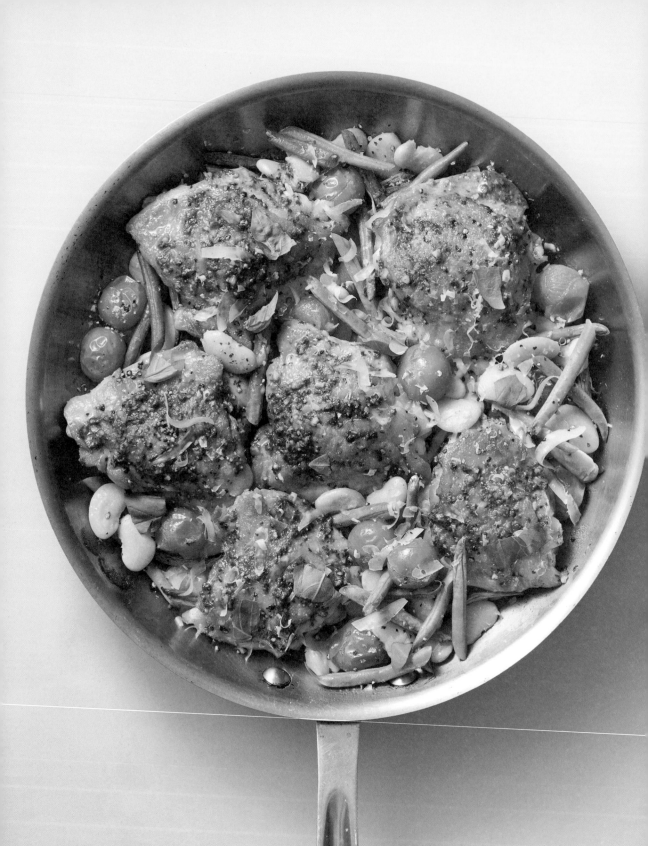

Skillet Pesto Chicken & Beans

This complete, hearty meal is cooked in one pan, making cleanup a breeze.

PREP: 10 MINUTES   TOTAL: 25 MINUTES

8 small chicken thighs (about 1½ pounds)

Kosher salt and ground black pepper

1 tablespoon olive oil

8 ounces green beans, halved

1 cup cherry tomatoes

1 (15-ounce) can butter beans, rinsed and drained

2 tablespoons store-bought or Homemade Pesto

Grated Parmesan cheese and chopped basil, for topping

1. Preheat the oven to 425°F. Season the chicken thighs with salt and pepper.

2. In a large oven-safe skillet, heat the oil on medium-high. Add the chicken, skin side down, and cook until the skin is golden brown, about 6 minutes.

3. Turn the chicken over; add the green beans, cherry tomatoes, and butter beans and season with ¼ teaspoon salt. Place the skillet in the oven and roast until chicken is cooked through (165°F), 12 to 15 minutes.

4. Brush the pesto over the chicken and top with grated Parmesan and chopped basil.

SERVES 4: About 450 calories, 38g protein, 22g carbohydrates, 26g fat (7g saturated), 6g fiber, 770mg sodium.

HOMEMADE PESTO

In a food processor or blender, pulse **3 cups loosely packed basil**, **1 large clove garlic** crushed with press, **½ cup extra-virgin olive oil**, **¼ cup grated Parmesan cheese**, **¼ cup toasted pine nuts**, **2 teaspoons fresh lemon juice**, and **¼ teaspoon ground black pepper** until smooth. Scoop into a covered container and refrigerate up to 3 days or freeze up to 3 months. Makes ¾ cup.

Roasted Baby Vine Tomato Grilled Chicken

Roasting cherry tomatoes brings out their natural sweetness and makes them—dare we say—addictive. See photo on page 8.

PREP: 20 MINUTES   TOTAL: 45 MINUTES

2 pounds mixed-size cherry tomatoes, on the vine if desired (about 4 pints)

4 large garlic cloves, crushed with a garlic press

¼ cup plus 1 tablespoon extra-virgin olive oil

¼ teaspoon crushed red pepper

Kosher salt

1½ pounds chicken breast cutlets, about ⅓-inch thick

Ground black pepper

1½ tablespoons chopped fresh tarragon

1. Preheat the oven to 500°F. Preheat the grill to medium-high. Cut about 1 cup of the largest tomatoes in half. On a rimmed baking sheet, toss all of the tomatoes with the garlic, ¼ cup of the oil, crushed red pepper, and ¾ teaspoon salt.

2. Roast the tomatoes on the upper oven rack, stirring halfway through, until the tomatoes burst and soften and some are beginning to char, about 20 minutes. (If most juices have evaporated, stir in 1 to 2 tablespoons water to create more sauce.)

3. Meanwhile, coat the chicken cutlets with the remaining 1 tablespoon of oil and season with ¼ teaspoon each salt and pepper. Grill until lightly charred and just cooked through (165°F), 2 to 3 minutes per side.

4. Gently toss the roasted tomatoes with the chopped tarragon. Spoon the tomatoes and any juices on top of the chicken and serve.

SERVES 4: About 390 calories, 37g protein, 10g carbohydrates, 22g fat (4g saturated), 2g fiber, 595mg sodium.

Harissa Grilled Chicken Kebabs

Glazed with a harissa pepper sauce, these chicken kebab skewers are a cut above the rest.

PREP: 10 MINUTES   **TOTAL: 20 MINUTES**

¼ cup harissa pepper paste

2 tablespoons extra-virgin olive oil

2 tablespoons honey

1¼ pounds skinless, boneless chicken breasts, thinly sliced

1 (15-ounce) can chickpeas, rinsed and drained

1 cup quick-cooking bulgur, cooked as the label directs

¾ cup finely chopped fresh parsley

Salt

1. Preheat the grill to medium-high.

2. In a large bowl, whisk the harissa with the oil and honey; set half aside for serving.

3. To the remaining harissa mixture, add the chicken breasts, tossing to coat; thread the chicken onto skewers. Grill until cooked through (165°F), about 6 minutes, turning once.

4. Toss the chickpeas with the cooked bulgur, parsley, and ½ teaspoon salt. Serve the chicken over the bulgur with the reserved harissa sauce alongside.

SERVES 4: About 495 calories, 39g protein, 57g carbohydrates, 13g fat (2g saturated), 13g fiber, 560mg sodium.

TIP

Harissa is a versatile spicy and aromatic chile paste used in North African and Middle Eastern cooking. It can be found in specialty grocery stores or online.

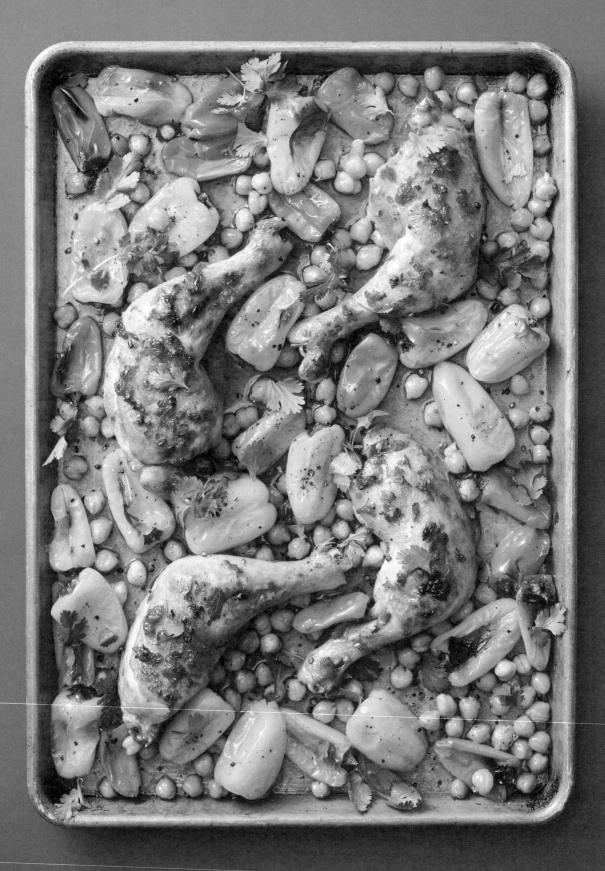

Sheet Pan Chickpea Chicken

You're just five key ingredients away from this smoky, Spanish-inspired one-pan dinner.

PREP: **5 MINUTES**   TOTAL: **35 MINUTES**

1 (15-ounce) can chickpeas, rinsed and drained

1 (16-ounce) bag mini sweet peppers

2 tablespoons olive oil

Salt and ground black pepper

2 tablespoons harissa pepper paste

4 small skin-on chicken legs (about 2½ pounds)

Chopped fresh cilantro, for serving

1. Preheat the oven to 425°F. On a large rimmed baking sheet, toss the chickpeas and sweet peppers with 1 tablespoon of the oil and ¼ teaspoon each salt and pepper.

2. In a small bowl, whisk together the harissa and the remaining 1 tablespoon oil. Rub the chicken with the harissa mixture. Nestle the chicken among the chickpeas and sweet peppers on the baking sheet and roast until the chicken is golden brown and cooked through (165°F), 20 to 25 minutes.

3. Toss with the cilantro before serving.

SERVES 4: About 630 calories, 39g protein, 22g carbohydrates, 42g fat (10g saturated), 6g fiber, 600mg sodium.

Chicken Marsala

This mushroom-studded chicken dish can be made in 30 minutes.

PREP: 5 MINUTES   TOTAL: 30 MINUTES

4 (6-ounce) boneless, skinless
    chicken breasts

Kosher salt and ground black pepper

3 tablespoons all-purpose flour

2 tablespoons olive oil

1 (10-ounce) package sliced cremini
    mushrooms

1 large shallot, finely chopped

1 clove garlic, finely chopped

½ cup low-sodium chicken broth

½ cup Marsala wine

1. Using the flat-side of a meat mallet or the bottom of a heavy saucepan, pound the chicken breasts to ½-inch thickness. Season with ¼ teaspoon each salt and pepper. Lightly coat the chicken breasts with the flour. Heat 1 tablespoon of the oil in a large skillet on medium and cook chicken until golden brown, 4 to 5 minutes per side; transfer to a plate.

2. Add the remaining 1 tablespoon oil to the same skillet. Cook the sliced mushrooms on medium-high, tossing occasionally, until golden brown, 5 minutes. Add the shallot and garlic. Season with ¼ teaspoon each salt and pepper; cook 2 minutes.

3. Add the broth and Marsala wine to the skillet, along with the browned chicken and its juices, and simmer until the liquid is reduced by half, about 4 minutes. Sprinkle with chopped parsley.

SERVES 4: About 335 calories, 42g protein, 14g carbohydrates, 12g fat (2g saturated), 1g fiber, 335mg sodium.

> **TIP**
>
> Serve this dish with sautéed spinach, if desired.

Chicken Souvlaki Skewers

Bring a traditional Greek meal—starring garlicky grape tomatoes and chicken kebabs—to your backyard with the help of your grill. See photo on page 11.

See photo on page 11.

PREP: 15 MINUTES   TOTAL: 25 MINUTES

1 pound skinless, boneless chicken breasts, cut into 1-inch chunks

3 tablespoons olive oil

½ teaspoon ground coriander

½ teaspoon dried oregano

Kosher salt and ground black pepper

1 pint grape tomatoes

2 cloves garlic, chopped

3 tablespoons fresh lemon juice

½ head romaine lettuce, shredded

4 green onions, thinly sliced

½ cup dill, chopped

4 whole-grain pitas, warmed

Lemon wedges, for serving

1. Preheat the grill to medium-high. Toss the chicken with 1 tablespoon of the olive oil, the coriander, oregano, and ¼ teaspoon each salt and pepper. Thread onto skewers.

2. Place the tomatoes and garlic on a large piece of heavy-duty aluminum foil. Drizzle with 1 tablespoon of the oil and sprinkle with ¼ teaspoon each salt and pepper. Fold and crimp the foil to form a sealed pouch.

3. Place the pouch and skewers on the hot grill. Cook, shaking the pouch and turning the skewers occasionally, until the chicken is cooked through (165°F), 8 to 10 minutes. Just before removing them from the grill, brush the chicken with 1 tablespoon of the lemon juice.

4. Meanwhile, in a salad bowl, toss the lettuce, green onions, and dill with the remaining 2 tablespoons lemon juice, 1 tablespoon oil, and ¼ teaspoon each salt and pepper.

5. Serve the chicken, tomatoes, and salad with pitas and lemon wedges.

SERVES 4: About 415 calories, 30g protein, 42g carbohydrates, 14g fat (2g saturated), 5g fiber, 750mg sodium.

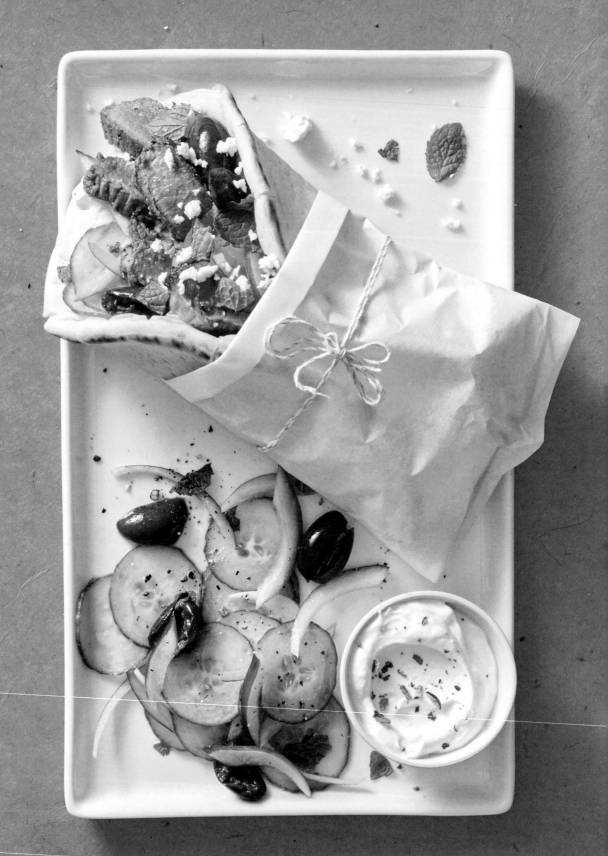

Lamb Souvlaki with Cucumber-Mint Salad

Kalamata olives and thick yogurt are the keys
to this Greek speciality. *Opa!*

PREP: **10 MINUTES**   TOTAL: **20 MINUTES**

1 pound lamb leg steak

1 tablespoon plus 2 teaspoons olive oil

½ teaspoon dried oregano

½ teaspoon ground coriander

Salt and ground black pepper

½ small red onion, thinly sliced

**½ English (seedless) cucumber,
very thinly sliced**

**¼ cup pitted Kalamata olives,
roughly chopped**

1 tablespoon red wine vinegar

½ cup plain Greek yogurt

4 whole-grain flatbreads, warmed

**Crumbled feta and fresh mint,
for serving**

1. Rub the lamb with 1 tablespoon of the oil, then season with the oregano, coriander, and ½ teaspoon each salt and pepper. Cook in a grill pan or a skillet on medium-high heat to the desired doneness, 2 to 3 minutes per side for medium-rare. Transfer to a cutting board and let rest 5 minutes before cutting the lamb into small cubes.

2. Meanwhile, in a bowl, toss the onion, cucumber, and olives with the vinegar and the remaining 2 teaspoons oil.

3. Spread about 2 tablespoons of Greek yogurt onto each warm flatbread. Top with lamb, cucumber salad, feta, and mint.

SERVES 4: About 500 calories, 32g protein, 46g carbohydrates, 21g fat (8g saturated), 3g fiber, 990mg sodium.

Moroccan Chicken with Preserved Lemons & Olives

You can buy pitted olives, but we think that unpitted olives are more flavorful. To split them open, press down hard on the olive with the flat side of a chef's knife. Remove the pit and you're good to go!

PREP: **25 MINUTES** TOTAL: **50 MINUTES**

- 2 tablespoons olive oil
- 8 small chicken thighs (about 1½ pounds)
- Kosher salt and ground black pepper
- 1 onion, thinly sliced
- 2 cloves garlic, finely chopped
- 1 teaspoon ground cumin
- 1 teaspoon ground cinnamon
- ½ teaspoon ground coriander
- ½ teaspoon ground ginger
- 1 cup low-sodium chicken broth
- ½ cup pitted small green olives
- ½ cup dried apricots, halved
- 2 tablespoons chopped preserved lemon (see right)
- ¼ cup flat-leaf parsley, chopped, and sliced toasted almonds, for serving (optional)

1. Preheat the oven to 425°F. Heat the oil in a large oven-safe skillet on medium. Season the chicken with ½ teaspoon each salt and pepper and cook, skin side down, until golden brown and crisp, 10 minutes. Flip and cook 1 minute more; transfer to a plate and cover to keep warm.

2. Add the onion to the skillet and cook, covered, stirring occasionally, until tender, 8 minutes. Uncover and stir in the garlic, cumin, cinnamon, coriander, ginger, and ½ teaspoon each salt and pepper. Cook, stirring occasionally, until onion is golden brown, 5 to 6 minutes more.

3. Stir in the broth, scraping up any browned bits. Return the chicken and any juices to the skillet along with the olives, apricots, and preserved lemon. Transfer to the oven and roast until the chicken is cooked through (165°F), 8 to 10 minutes.

4. Sprinkle with parsley and almonds, if desired, and serve.

SERVES 4: About 605 calories, 38g protein, 10g carbohydrates, 46g fat (11g saturated), 3g fiber, 985mg sodium.

PRESERVED LEMONS

Bring a covered 6-quart saucepot of water to boiling on high heat. With tongs, place a 1-quart widemouthed glass canning jar and metal lid into the boiling water. Boil 2 minutes, turning occasionally. Remove and invert onto a clean kitchen towel to dry. Scrub **5 small lemons**, trim the ends, and quarter them lengthwise, leaving ¼ inch of the bottoms intact. For each lemon, rub **1 tablespoon salt** between the quarters; place in the canning jar. Add enough **fresh lemon juice** to cover the lemons completely (about 1½ cups). Cover with the lid. Let stand at least 4 weeks in a cool spot. Refrigerate after opening for up to 6 months.

Chicken Cacciatore

Bring on the veggies in this healthy chicken dish. Serve
with a side of whole-grain pasta, if desired.

PREP: 25 MINUTES   TOTAL: 50 MINUTES

2 tablespoons olive oil

6 small (5-ounce) boneless, skinless
chicken breasts

Kosher salt and ground black pepper

1 (10-ounce) package cremini mushrooms,
quartered

1 small onion, thinly sliced

1 red bell pepper, seeded and thinly sliced

2 cloves garlic, finely chopped

2 teaspoons fresh rosemary,
finely chopped

1 bay leaf

¾ cup dry white wine

1 (28-ounce) can diced tomatoes

8 ounces kale, stems discarded and
leaves chopped

½ cup pitted green olives

¼ cup flat-leaf parsley, chopped

1. Heat the oil in a large deep skillet on medium-high. Season the chicken with ½ teaspoon each salt and pepper and cook until golden brown, 3 to 4 minutes per side; transfer to a plate and cover to keep warm.

2. Add the mushrooms to the skillet and cook, tossing occasionally, until golden brown and tender, about 4 minutes. Transfer to the plate with the chicken.

3. Lower the heat to medium and add the onion, bell pepper, garlic, rosemary, and bay leaf. Cook, stirring occasionally, until tender, 8 to 10 minutes. Add the wine and cook, stirring and scraping up any browned bits, until reduced by half, about 3 minutes. Stir in tomatoes and their juices.

4. Return the chicken and mushrooms to the skillet, nestling the chicken in the tomatoes, and simmer, covered, for 15 minutes. Fold in the kale and cook, covered, 10 to 12 minutes more. Uncover, discard the bay leaf, stir in the olives and parsley, and serve.

SERVES 6: About 300 calories, 36g protein, 15g carbohydrates, 10g fat (2g saturated), 3g fiber, 690mg sodium.

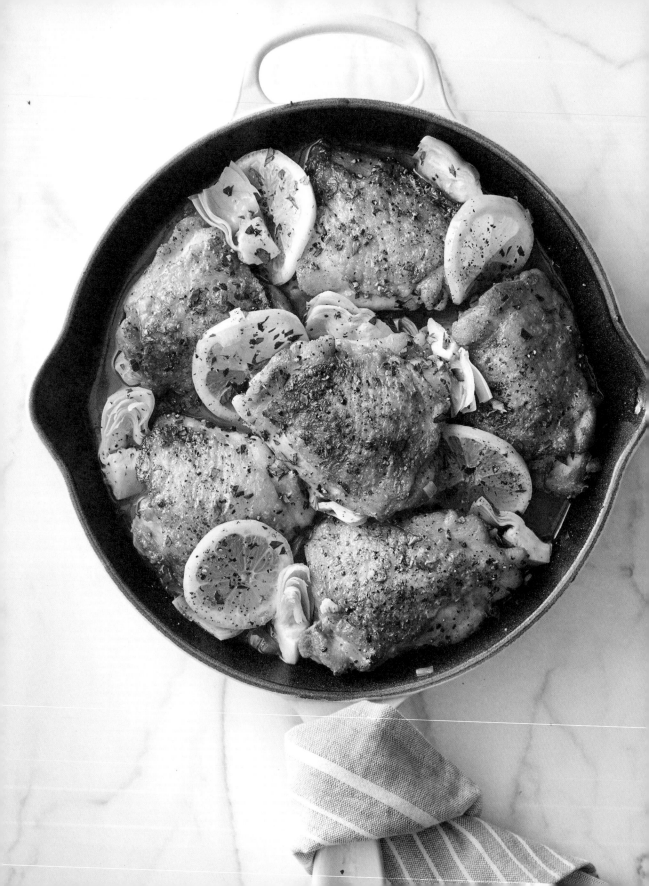

Skillet Lemon Chicken with Artichokes

Lemony artichokes pair perfectly with crispy, golden chicken thighs.

PREP: **20 MINUTES** TOTAL: **30 MINUTES**

1 tablespoon plus 1 teaspoon olive oil

6 small chicken thighs (about 2 pounds)

Salt and ground black pepper

1 medium onion, finely chopped

⅔ cup dry white wine

1 (14-ounce) can artichoke hearts, rinsed, drained, and quartered

1 lemon, thinly sliced crosswise, seeds removed

½ bunch fresh parsley, chopped

1½ cups brown rice, cooked as the label directs

1. Preheat the oven to 425°F. Line a large rimmed baking sheet with aluminum foil.

2. In a 12-inch skillet, heat 1 teaspoon of the oil on medium-high heat. Season the chicken thighs with ½ teaspoon each salt and pepper. Cook the chicken in the skillet, skin side down, until golden brown, 5 to 8 minutes. Remove from the heat.

3. Transfer the chicken, skin side up, to the prepared baking sheet. Roast the chicken in the oven until cooked through (165°F), 12 to 15 minutes.

4. Meanwhile, start the sauce. Return the skillet to medium heat and add the chopped onion. Season with ¼ teaspoon salt and cook, stirring occasionally, for 3 minutes. Add the white wine and bring to a simmer. Let simmer, scraping up any browned bits in the pan, for 2 minutes. Stir the remaining 1 tablespoon oil into the skillet. Add the artichoke hearts and lemon slices.

5. Spoon the sauce over the cooked chicken and sprinkle with the chopped parsley. Serve with the brown rice.

SERVES 4: About 510 calories, 34g protein, 10g carbohydrates, 36g fat (11g saturated), 1g fiber, 790mg sodium.

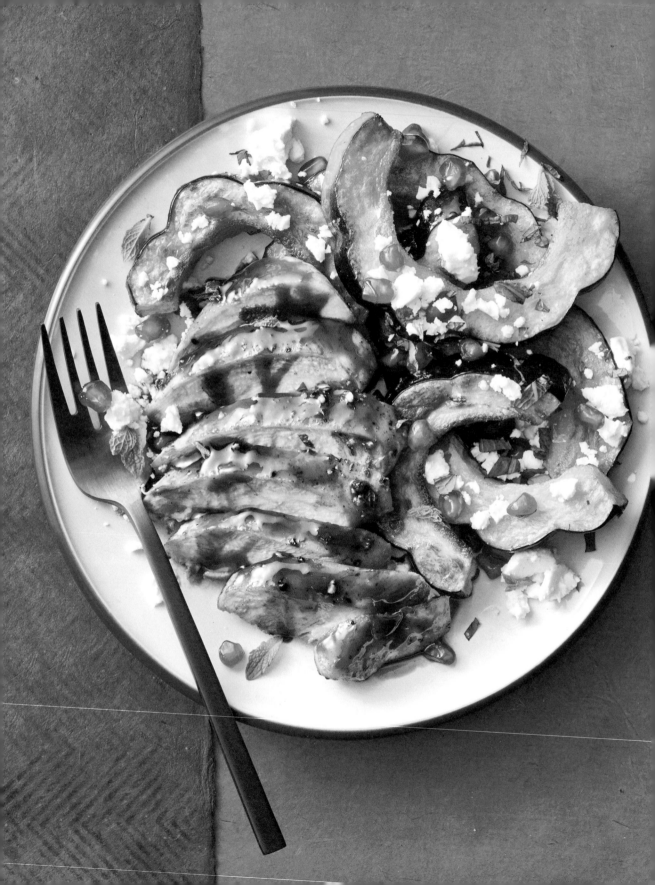

Pomegranate-Honey-Glazed Chicken & Squash

Mix the hottest flavors of the harvest season
into this heart-healthy chicken dish.

PREP: 20 MINUTES   TOTAL: 35 MINUTES

1 medium acorn squash (about 1½ pounds)

2 tablespoons olive oil

Kosher salt

Pinch of cayenne pepper

4 (6-ounce) boneless, skinless
  chicken breasts

Ground black pepper

⅓ cup pomegranate juice

¼ cup honey

1 tablespoon balsamic vinegar

⅓ cup crumbled feta cheese

⅓ cup pomegranate seeds

1 bunch fresh mint, finely chopped

1. Preheat the oven to 425°F. Remove the seeds from the squash and cut it crosswise into ¾-inch-thick slices.

2. On a large rimmed baking sheet, toss the squash slices with 1 tablespoon of the oil, ½ teaspoon salt, and the cayenne pepper. Roast until golden brown and tender, 20 to 25 minutes.

3. Meanwhile, heat the remaining 1 tablespoon oil in a large skillet on medium-high. Season the chicken breasts with ½ teaspoon salt and ¼ teaspoon pepper. Add to the skillet and sauté until golden brown and cooked through (165°F), 6 to 8 minutes per side. Remove the chicken from the skillet and set it aside.

4. Return the skillet to medium heat, add the pomegranate juice, and cook, scraping up any browned bits, for 1 minute. Add the honey and balsamic vinegar and cook until thick and syrupy, 3 to 5 minutes.

5. Brush the chicken with the glaze. Sprinkle the squash with the crumbled feta, pomegranate seeds, and chopped mint before serving alongside the chicken.

SERVES 4: About 440 calories, 42g protein, 38g carbohydrates, 14g fat (4g saturated), 6g fiber, 680mg sodium.

Chicken Quinoa Bowls

We'll take this warm quinoa and arugula bowl, topped with herb-crusted chicken, olives, and tomatoes, for lunch any and every day.

PREP: 15 MINUTES   **TOTAL: 20 MINUTES**

4 (5-ounce) chicken breast cutlets

¼ teaspoon herbes de Provence

Salt and ground black pepper

¼ cup Champagne vinegar

¼ cup olive oil

2 green onions

2 tablespoons Dijon mustard

1 cup red quinoa, cooked as the label directs

4 cups packed arugula

12 ounces (¾ pint) grape tomatoes, halved

⅔ cup pitted green olives, quartered

1. Preheat the grill to medium-high.

2. Season the chicken cutlets with the herbes de Provence and ¼ teaspoon each salt and pepper. Grill until cooked through (165°F), 3 minutes per side.

3. In a blender, puree the Champagne vinegar, oil, green onions, mustard, and ¼ teaspoon salt. In a large bowl, toss half the vinaigrette with the cooked quinoa, arugula, grape tomatoes, and green olives. Serve the chicken over the quinoa with the remaining vinaigrette.

SERVES 4: About 500 calories, 36g protein, 35g carbohydrates, 23g fat (4g saturated), 8g fiber, 865mg sodium.

Grilled Lamb & Artichoke Kebabs

Drizzle lemon juice over grilled lamb to cut the meaty flavor and for some added tang.

PREP: 1 HOUR **TOTAL:** 1 HOUR 30 MINUTES

2½ pounds boneless lamb leg, trimmed and cut into 1-inch chunks

2 tablespoons olive oil

1 teaspoon ground coriander

1 teaspoon dried oregano

Kosher salt and ground black pepper

3 lemons

2 cloves garlic, finely chopped

¼ cup flat-leaf parsley, chopped

16 large marinated artichoke hearts

2 bunches green onions

1. In a large bowl, toss the lamb with the oil, coriander, oregano, and ½ teaspoon each salt and pepper. Finely grate the zest of 2 lemons over the lamb; add the garlic and parsley and toss to combine. Cover and let sit 1 hour or refrigerate overnight.

2. Meanwhile, cut all the lemons and artichoke hearts in half; cut the green onions crosswise into 2½-inch pieces.

3. Preheat the grill or a grill pan on medium-high. Thread the artichoke hearts, green onions, and lamb onto skewers.

4. Grill the kebabs, turning occasionally, until the lamb reaches the desired doneness, 6 to 8 minutes for medium-rare. Grill the lemons, cut sides down, until charred, 2 to 3 minutes. Squeeze the lemons over the kebabs and serve.

SERVES 8: About 265 calories, 28g protein, 8g carbohydrates, 15g fat (4g saturated), 2g fiber, 320mg sodium.

TIP

Large metal skewers are the best for kebabs. Choose skewers with flat shafts rather than rounded ones; food will be less likely to slip or spin around as you turn the skewers.

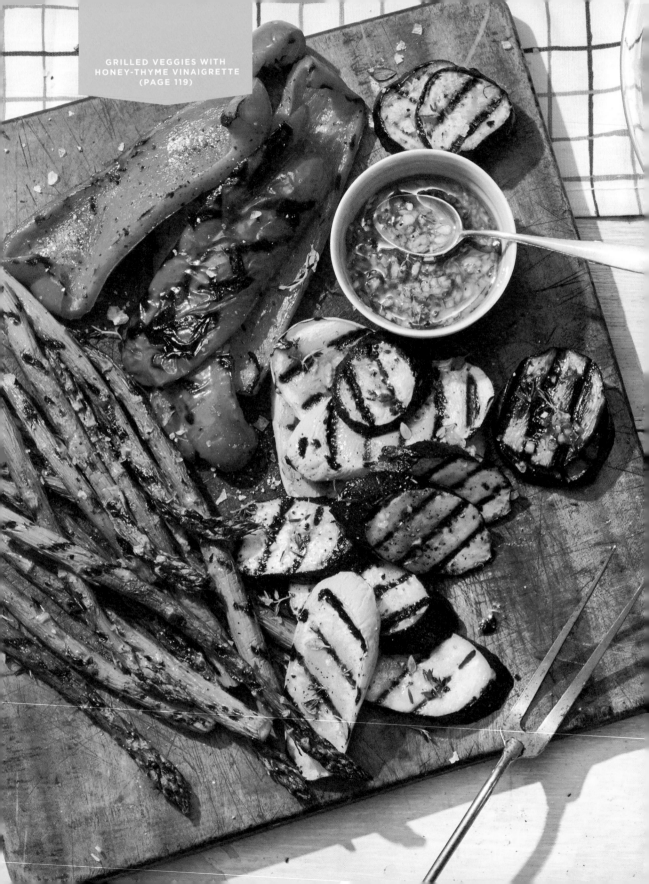

GRILLED VEGGIES WITH
HONEY-THYME VINAIGRETTE
(PAGE 119)

5 | Meatless Meals & Vegetables

Vegetables are a main component of the Mediterranean diet. In this chapter, you will find meatless mains chock-full of whole grains and healthy vegetables that will keep you feeling full. Also included are sides that can accompany any healthy meal. With a variety of vegetables and seasonings, there is surely something here you will love. Plus, dishes with Moroccan flavors, Provençal tastes, and more will transport you to far-off places without ever having to leave your kitchen.

Quinoa-Stuffed Acorn Squash with Cranberries & Feta 111

Summer Squash Frittata 112

Heirloom Tomato Salad 113

Lemony Asparagus, Beans & Peas 114

Marinated Mushrooms 115

Green Beans with Olive-Almond Tapenade 117

Moroccan Carrots 118

Grilled Veggies with Honey-Thyme Vinaigrette 119

Spinach & Artichoke Squash Casserole 121

White Bean & Broccolini Salad 123

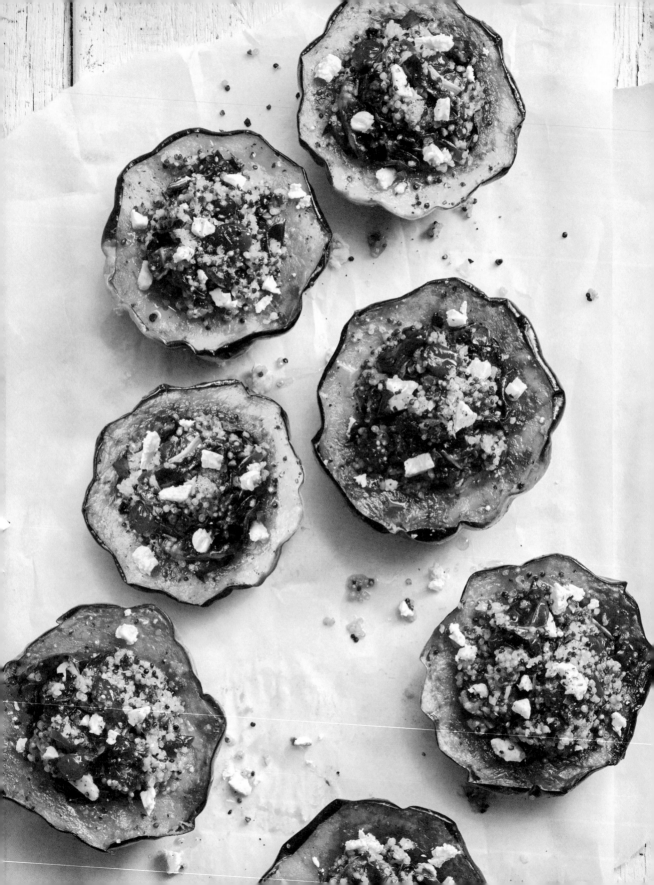

Quinoa-Stuffed Acorn Squash with Cranberries & Feta

Packed with antioxidant-rich cranberries, Swiss chard, and 100 percent whole grains, this vegetarian main is hefty enough to keep you satisfied, and it's good for your heart too.

PREP: 10 MINUTES   **TOTAL: 45 MINUTES**

- **4 small acorn squashes (about 4½ pounds)**
- **3 tablespoons olive oil**
- **Salt and ground black pepper**
- **1 medium onion, finely chopped**
- **2 cloves garlic, finely chopped**
- **1 cup mixed-color quinoa**
- **2 teaspoons fresh thyme leaves**
- **2 cups water**
- **⅓ cup dried cranberries**
- **1 small bunch Swiss chard, stems discarded and leaves roughly chopped (about 6 cups)**
- **Crumbled feta cheese, for serving (optional)**

1. Place a rimmed baking sheet in the oven and preheat it to 425°F. From each squash, cut ½ inch from the pointy end (this will help them stand up straight), then halve each one through its center; spoon out and discard the seeds. Rub the squashes with 1 tablespoon of the oil and season with ¼ teaspoon each salt and pepper. Arrange the squash halves, hollow sides down, on the baking sheet and roast until tender, 25 to 30 minutes.

2. Meanwhile, in a 3- to 4-quart saucepan, heat the remaining 2 tablespoons oil on medium. Add the onion and ½ teaspoon each salt and pepper. Cook, covered, for 7 minutes, stirring often. Stir in the garlic; cook 2 minutes.

3. Add the quinoa to the saucepan and toss to coat, then add the thyme and water; simmer, covered, 10 minutes. Stir in the cranberries; simmer, covered, 5 minutes.

4. Remove the saucepan from the heat; place the Swiss chard on top of the quinoa and cover the pan with a clean dish towel, followed by the lid. Let stand 10 minutes.

5. Transfer the squash to a platter, hollow sides up. Fold the chard into the quinoa, then spoon the mixture into the squash halves. Top with feta, if desired.

SERVES 8: About 260 calories, 5g protein, 49g carbohydrates, 7g fat (1g saturated), 10g fiber, 255mg sodium.

Summer Squash Frittata

Your favorite summer vegetable gives this cheesy frittata a pop of color.

PREP: 10 MINUTES   TOTAL: 35 MINUTES

1½ pounds summer squash

Salt

8 large eggs

4 ounces Gruyère cheese, shredded

¾ cup milk

2 green onions, thinly sliced

1. Preheat the oven to 375°F.

2. Thinly slice the summer squash. In a colander, toss the summer squash with ¼ teaspoon salt and let stand 10 minutes. Gently squeeze the summer squash until very dry.

3. Meanwhile, in a bowl, whisk together the eggs, Gruyère, milk, and green onions.

4. Heat a 10-inch oven-safe skillet on medium. Add the egg mixture and stir in the squash. Cook, stirring occasionally and pulling back the edges, until the bottom begins to set, about 2 minutes. Cook, without stirring, for 3 minutes.

5. Transfer the skillet to the oven and bake until set, 20 to 25 minutes.

SERVES 4: About 320 calories, 25g protein, 9g carbohydrates, 21g fat (10g saturated), 2g fiber, 690mg sodium.

Heirloom Tomato Salad

Basil packs an herbaceous punch in this light and
refreshing side salad. See photo on page 122.

See photo on page 122.

TOTAL: 15 MINUTES

¼ cup extra-virgin olive oil

2 tablespoons champagne vinegar

1 teaspoon honey

Kosher salt

Pepper

1 pint mixed-color cherry or grape
tomatoes, halved

2 tablespoons finely chopped chives,
plus more for serving

1 pound heirloom tomatoes, some sliced
and some cut into wedges

Small basil leaves, for serving

1. In a medium bowl, whisk together the oil,
vinegar, honey, and ½ teaspoon each salt and
pepper. Add the cherry tomatoes and the
chives and toss to combine.

2. Arrange the heirloom tomatoes on a plate
and sprinkle with ¼ teaspoon each salt and
pepper. Spoon the cherry tomato mixture on
top. Top the dish with additional chives and
basil leaves to serve.

SERVES 6: About 105 calories, 1g protein,
6g carbohydrates, 10g fat (2g saturated), 1g fiber,
185mg sodium.

Lemony Asparagus, Beans & Peas

Don't skip the sesame seeds in this green beans, asparagus, and peas medley—they really make the dish special.

PREP: 20 MINUTES   TOTAL: 40 MINUTES

Salt

1½ pounds thin asparagus, cut into thirds on an angle

12 ounces haricots verts or green beans, trimmed

8 ounces fresh or frozen (thawed) peas

4 tablespoons olive oil

1 large onion, very thinly sliced

¼ cup fresh lemon juice

1 tablespoon snipped fresh chives

1 tablespoon sesame seeds

2 teaspoons honey

1 clove garlic, crushed with a garlic press

Ground black pepper

1. Heat a covered 7- to 8-quart saucepot of salted water to boiling on high. To a large bowl, add about 6 cups ice; fill it with cold water. Add asparagus, haricots verts, and peas to the boiling water. Boil until asparagus and haricots verts are tender, 5 to 7 minutes. Drain well, then immediately add them to the bowl of ice water. Let stand until the vegetables are cold, then drain well.

2. In a 10-inch skillet, heat 1 tablespoon of the oil on medium. Add the onion and a pinch of salt. Cook until the onion is tender and deep golden brown, 12 to 15 minutes, stirring frequently. Set aside.

3. In a small bowl, whisk together the lemon juice, chives, sesame seeds, honey, garlic, ¾ teaspoon salt, ½ teaspoon pepper, and the remaining 3 tablespoons oil.

4. To serve, toss the vegetables with the onions and vinaigrette.

SERVES 10: About 105 calories, 4g protein, 11g carbohydrates, 6g fat (1g saturated), 4g fiber, 210mg sodium.

Marinated Mushrooms

Dress up a boring sandwich or salad with these sweet
and tangy mushrooms. Or serve them as tapas the next time
you entertain. See the photo on page 122.

See the photo on page 122.

PREP: 10 MINUTES   TOTAL: 1 HOUR

½ cup extra-virgin olive oil

3 tablespoons white wine vinegar

2 tablespoons fresh lemon juice

1 tablespoon maple syrup

2 tablespoons chopped flat-leaf parsley

2 tablespoons chopped dill

Kosher salt and ground black pepper

1 pound cremini mushrooms, thinly sliced

1. In a large bowl, whisk together the oil, vinegar, lemon juice, maple syrup, parsley, dill, and ½ teaspoon each salt and pepper. Add the mushrooms and gently toss to combine.

2. Let the mixture sit at room temperature, tossing occasionally, until the mushrooms are tender, at least 1 hour. Transfer to jars and store in the refrigerator for up to 3 days.

SERVES 8: About 35 calories, 1g protein,
3g carbohydrates, 3g fat (1g saturated),
0g fiber, 25mg sodium.

MOROCCAN CARROTS (page 118)

GREEN BEANS WITH OLIVE-ALMOND TAPENADE

Green Beans with Olive-Almond Tapenade

Give green beans a Provençal flavor with an almond, olive, parsley, and lemon zest tapenade.

PREP: 15 MINUTES   TOTAL: 25 MINUTES

¼ cup whole almonds, toasted

½ cup large pitted green olives

1 teaspoon grated lemon zest

3 tablespoons packed fresh parsley leaves, plus more for garnish

2 tablespoons extra-virgin olive oil

Salt and ground black pepper

1½ pounds green beans, trimmed

1. In a food processor, pulse the almonds until finely chopped. Add the olives, lemon zest, and parsley; pulse until finely ground, stopping and scraping down occasionally. Add the oil and pulse until well blended; season with ⅛ teaspoon salt and ¼ teaspoon pepper.

2. Heat a large covered pot of salted water to boiling on high. Add the green beans to the boiling water; cook until crisp-tender, about 4 minutes. Drain well; place in a serving bowl.

3. Add the tapenade to the beans and toss until evenly coated. Garnish with parsley. Serve warm or at room temperature.

SERVES 4: About 185 calories, 5g protein, 13g carbohydrates, 14g fat (2g saturated), 6g fiber, 380mg sodium.

Moroccan Carrots

Upgrade a traditional carrot side with cinnamon, sweet paprika, cumin, and harissa. See photo on page page 116.

PREP: 15 MINUTES   TOTAL: 20 MINUTES

3 large carrots, peeled and very thinly sliced

½ teaspoon ground cumin

½ teaspoon sweet paprika

Pinch of ground cinnamon

Pinch of cayenne pepper

2 tablespoons extra-virgin olive oil

1 tablespoon fresh lemon juice

1 small clove garlic, crushed with a garlic press

½ cup packed parsley leaves, coarsely chopped

2 teaspoons sesame seeds

Salt and ground black pepper

3 tablespoons harissa pepper paste (optional)

1. Place the carrots in a medium heatproof bowl.

2. In a small skillet, toast the cumin, paprika, cinnamon, and cayenne pepper on medium-low until fragrant, about 1 minute, stirring. Stir in the oil, then the lemon juice. Heat to a simmer. Add the garlic and cook until the mixture is very hot, 15 to 20 seconds.

3. Pour the hot dressing over the carrots; toss until evenly coated. Add the parsley, sesame seeds, ¼ teaspoon each salt and pepper, and harissa, if using; toss until combined. Serve at room temperature.

SERVES 4: About 105 calories, 1g protein, 7g carbohydrates, 8g fat (1g saturated), 2g fiber, 190mg sodium.

Grilled Veggies with Honey-Thyme Vinaigrette

Meet your new go-to summer side. This vinaigrette will be your new favorite. See photo on page 108.

PREP: **15 MINUTES**   TOTAL: **20 MINUTES**

2 tablespoons red wine vinegar

½ teaspoon honey

Kosher salt and ground black pepper

1 shallot, finely chopped

1 teaspoon fresh thyme, plus more (optional) for serving

2 yellow summer squash, sliced

2 zucchini, sliced

1 small eggplant, sliced

2 red bell peppers, seeded and quartered lengthwise

1 pound asparagus, trimmed

2 tablespoons olive oil, plus more for brushing vegetables

1. Preheat the grill to medium-high. In a small bowl, whisk together the vinegar, honey, and ½ teaspoon each salt and pepper to dissolve. Stir in the shallot and thyme; let sit while you grill the vegetables.

2. Brush the vegetables with oil and season with salt and pepper. Grill, turning once, until lightly charred and just tender, 2 to 4 minutes per side; transfer to a platter.

3. Stir the remaining 2 tablespoons oil into the vinegar mixture; serve over the vegetables and sprinkle with additional thyme, if desired.

SERVES 6: About 135 calories, 5g protein, 15g carbohydrates, 8g fat (1g saturated), 6g fiber, 250mg sodium.

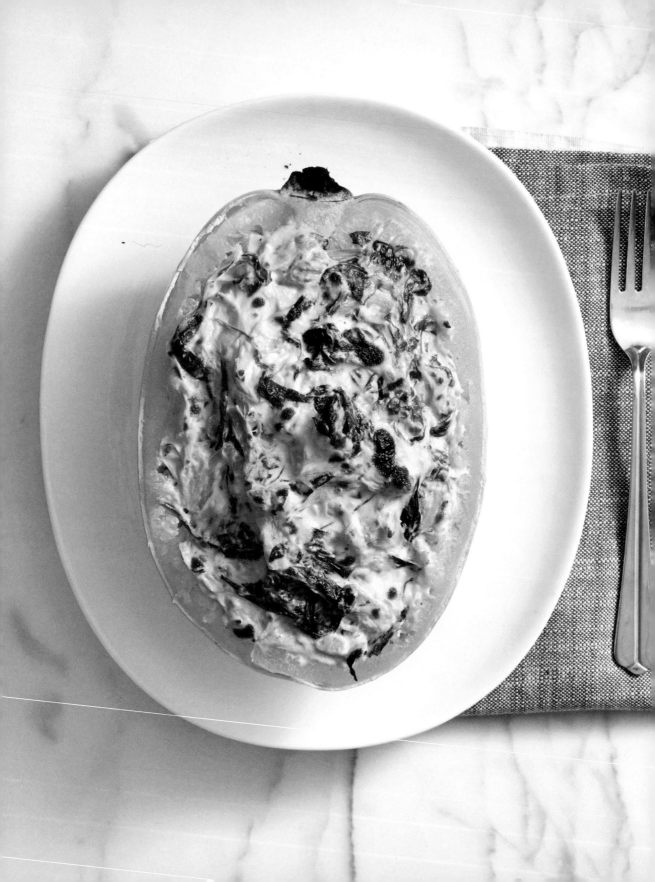

Spinach & Artichoke Squash Casserole

Serve spinach and artichokes, two staple appetizer ingredients,
in a hollowed spaghetti squash for a sophisticated side dish.

PREP: 20 MINUTES   TOTAL: 30 MINUTES

2 medium spaghetti squashes

1 medium shallot, finely chopped

1 tablespoon extra-virgin olive oil

6 cups packed spinach

Salt

8 ounces reduced-fat cream cheese, softened

1 cup drained marinated artichoke hearts, chopped

¼ cup grated Parmesan cheese

½ teaspoon lemon zest

Ground black pepper

1. Poke the spaghetti squashes all over with a knife; place them in a large microwave-safe dish. Cook on High for 10 minutes. Turn over; cook 10 minutes more or until a knife slips in easily.

2. Preheat the broiler to High.

3. In a 6-quart saucepot on medium heat, cook the shallot in the oil 3 minutes, stirring. Add the spinach and ¼ teaspoon salt; cook until wilted, about 2 minutes. Add the cream cheese, artichoke hearts, Parmesan, lemon zest, and ½ teaspoon pepper, stirring until the cheeses melts.

4. Cut the squashes into halves; discard the seeds. Using a fork, scrape the insides into strands; sprinkle with ⅛ teaspoon salt.

5. Divide the spinach mixture among the squash halves. Broil until browned, 3 to 4 minutes, and then serve immediately.

SERVES 4: About 325 calories, 11g protein, 25g carbohydrates, 22g fat (9g saturated), 6g fiber, 720mg sodium.

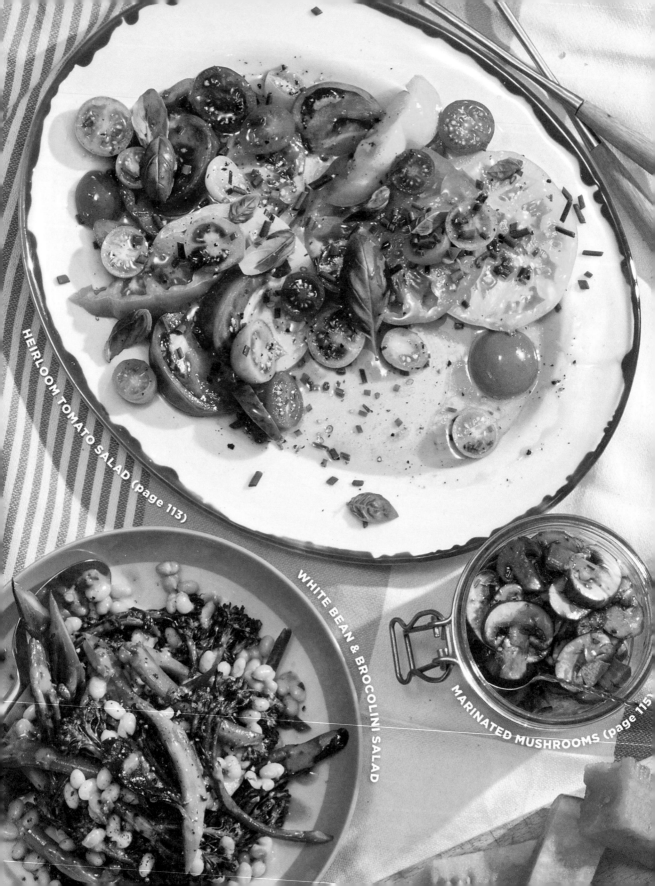

HEIRLOOM TOMATO SALAD (page 113)

WHITE BEAN & BROCOLINI SALAD

MARINATED MUSHROOMS (page 115)

White Bean & Broccolini Salad

Honey mustard and crushed red pepper flakes give this veggie salad a unique sweet and spicy flavor.

TOTAL: 20 MINUTES

Kosher salt

1 pound Broccolini, trimmed (about 3 bunches)

3 tablespoons olive oil

1 teaspoon lemon zest

2 tablespoons fresh lemon juice

2 tablespoons honey mustard

½ teaspoon crushed red pepper

Ground black pepper

2 tablespoons capers, drained and chopped

1 (15.5-ounce) can small white beans, rinsed and drained

1. In a large pot of salted boiling water, cook the Broccolini until the stalks are crisp-tender, about 2 minutes. Drain and transfer to an ice bath to cool. Drain well and pat dry, then cut the Broccolini into large pieces.

2. In a large bowl, whisk together the oil, lemon zest and juice, honey mustard, crushed red pepper, and ¼ teaspoon each salt and pepper; stir in the capers. Add the Broccolini and white beans and toss to coat.

SERVES 6: About 145 calories, 6g protein, 19g carbohydrates, 8g fat (1g saturated), 6g fiber, 375mg sodium.

TIP

An ice bath is an easy way to quickly stop the cooking process or safely cool food. To create one, fill a large bowl with ice and cold water. Place the container with your food in the ice bath.

Index

Note: Page numbers in *italics* indicate photos separate from recipes.

Note: Page numbers in italics indicate photos separate from recipes.

A

Almonds
  Almond-Pepper Vinaigrette, 27
  Olive-Almond Tapenade, 117
Artichokes
  Grilled Lamb & Artichoke Kebabs, 107
  Roasted Artichokes with Caesar Dip, *28-29*
  Skillet Lemon Chicken with Artichokes, *102-103*
  Spinach & Artichoke Squash Casserole, *120-121*
Arugula Pesto Crostini, 19
Asparagus
  about: trimming and slicing, 35
  Grilled Veggies with Honey-Thyme Vinaigrette, *108*, 119
  Lemony Asparagus, Beans & Peas, 114
  Roasted Cumin Shrimp & Asparagus, *86-87*
  Spring Minestrone, *34-35*
  Spring Veggie & Goat Cheese Spaghetti, *62-63*
  Tahini-Lemon Quinoa with Asparagus Ribbons, *72-73*
Avocados, in Beet, Mushroom & Avocado Salad, *44-45*

B

Basil
  Cherry Tomato Casserole with White Beans & Basil, 71
  Creamy Basil Potato Salad, 66
  Homemade Pesto, 91
  Tomato-Basil Gnocchi, *52*, 58
Beans and other legumes. *See also* Green beans
  Cherry Tomato Casserole with White Beans & Basil, 71
  Homemade Hummus, 25
  Lentil Salad, 79
  Mediterranean Hummus Egg Smash, *12*, 25
  Sheet Pan Chickpea Chicken, *94-95*
  soups with. *See* Soups
  Tahini-Lemon Quinoa with Asparagus Ribbons, *72-73*
  White Bean & Broccolini Salad, *122-123*
Beet, Mushroom & Avocado Salad, *44-45*
Bok choy, soy-glazed cod and, *80-81*

Bowls, chicken quinoa, 106
Broccolini, in White Bean & Broccolini Salad, *122-123*
Butternut squash. *See* Squash

C

Caesar Dip, 29
Caper Gremolata, 70
Carrots
  Green Goddess Carrot Salad, *46-47*
  Moroccan Carrots, *116*, 118
Cauliflower
  Cauliflower Soup, 38
  Kale & Roasted Cauliflower Salad, *50-51*
Cheese
  Arugula Pesto Crostini, 19
  Feta-Dill Greek Caesar, *32*, 49
  Grilled Leek, Zucchini & Ricotta Pizza, *16-17*
  Quinoa-Stuffed Acorn Squash with Cranberries & Feta, *110-111*
  Spinach & Gruyère Potato Casserole, *68-69*
  Spring Veggie & Goat Cheese Spaghetti, *62-63*
  Tomato-Basil Gnocchi, *52*, 58
Cherry Tomato Casserole with White Beans & Basil, 71
Cherry tomatoes. *See* Tomatoes
Chicken
  Creamy Lemon Chicken Pasta, *60-61*
  Lemon-Dill Chicken Meatball Soup, 39
Chicken main dishes
  about: overview of recipes, 75
  Chicken & Red Plum Salad, 88
  Chicken Cacciatore, 101
  Chicken Marsala, 96
  Chicken Quinoa Bowls, 106
  Chicken Souvlaki Skewers, 97
  Chipotle Orange Chicken, 89
  Harissa Grilled Chicken Kebabs, 93
  Moroccan Chicken with Preserved Lemons & Olives, 100
  Pomegranate-Honey-Glazed Chicken & Squash, *104-105*
  Roasted Baby Vine Tomato Grilled Chicken, 92
  Sheet Pan Chickpea Chicken, *94-95*
  Skillet Lemon Chicken with Artichokes, *102-103*
  Skillet Pesto Chicken & Beans, *90-91*
Chickpeas. *See* Beans and other legumes
Citrus
  Chipotle Orange Chicken, 89
  Creamy Lemon Chicken Pasta, *60-61*
  Lemon-Dill Chicken Meatball Soup, 39
  Lemony Asparagus, Beans & Peas, 114

Preserved Lemons, 100
  Skillet Lemon Chicken with Artichokes, *102-103*
  Tahini-Lemon Quinoa with Asparagus Ribbons, *72-73*
  Zesty Lemon-Herb Baked Flounder, 82
Couscous
  Roasted Cumin Shrimp & Asparagus, *86-87*
  Shrimp Packets with Kale Couscous, *84-85*
Cranberries, in Quinoa-Stuffed Acorn Squash with Cranberries & Feta, *110-111*
Creamy Basil Potato Salad, 66
Creamy Lemon Chicken Pasta, *60-61*
Creamy Spaghetti & Zoodles, *56-57*
Crispy Smashed Potatoes with Caper Gremolata, 70
Crostini, arugula pesto, 19
Cucumber-Mint Salad, *98-99*

E

Easiest-Ever Paella, *74*, 83
Eggplant
  Grilled Veggies with Honey-Thyme Vinaigrette, *108*, 119
  Plum Tomato & Eggplant Shakshuka, *30-31*
Eggs
  Mediterranean Hummus Egg Smash, *12*, 25
  Spanish Potato Omelet, 67
  Summer Squash Frittata, 112

F

Fennel, roasted, radicchio salad with shrimp and, 48
Feta. *See* Cheese
Fish. *See* Seafood references
Fruit, importance for Mediterranean diet, 11

G

Gnocchi, tomato-basil, *52*, 58
Grains, importance of whole-grains, 11. *See also* Couscous; Pasta and pasta alternatives; Quinoa; Rice
Greek Yellow Split Pea Dip, 18
Green beans
  Green Beans with Olive-Almond Tapenade, *116-117*
  Lemony Asparagus, Beans & Peas, 114
  Skillet Pesto Chicken & Beans, *90-91*
Green Goddess Carrot Salad, *46-47*
Grilled Lamb & Artichoke Kebabs, 107
Grilled Leek, Zucchini & Ricotta Pizza, *16-17*
Grilled Veggies with Honey-Thyme Vinaigrette, *108*, 119

H

Harissa Grilled Chicken Kebabs, 93
Heirloom Tomato Salad, 113, *122*
Honey-Ginger Cedar Plank Salmon, *76*–77
Honey-Soy-Glazed Salmon with Peppers, 78
Honey-Thyme Vinaigrette, 119
Hummus, *12*, 25

I

Indulgences (conscious), enjoying, 11

K

Kale
    Beet, Mushroom & Avocado Salad, 44–45
    Kale & Roasted Cauliflower Salad, *50*–51
    Shrimp Packets with Kale Couscous, *84*–85
Kebabs/skewers
    about: choosing skewers, 107
    Chicken Souvlaki Skewers, 97
    Grilled Lamb & Artichoke Kebabs, 107
    Harissa Grilled Chicken Kebabs, 93
    Swordfish Kebabs with Mint Pesto, 24

L

Lamb
    Grilled Lamb & Artichoke Kebabs, 107
    Lamb Souvlaki with Cucumber-Mint Salad, *98*–99
Leek, grilled, on pizza, *16*–17
Lemon. *See* Citrus
Lentils. *See* Beans and other legumes; Soups
Linguine. *See* Pasta and pasta alternatives

M

Main dishes, 75–107. *See also* Chicken main dishes; Meatless mains and sides; Seafood main dishes
    about: overview of recipes, 75
    Grilled Lamb & Artichoke Kebabs, 107
    Lamb Souvlaki with Cucumber-Mint Salad, *98*–99
Marinated Mushrooms, 115, *122*
Meatball soup, chicken, 39
Meatless mains and sides, 109–123. *See also* Salads
    about: overview of recipes, 109
    Green Beans with Olive-Almond Tapenade, *116*–117
    Grilled Veggies with Honey-Thyme Vinaigrette, *108*, 119
    Heirloom Tomato Salad, 113, *122*
    Lemony Asparagus, Beans & Peas, 114
    Marinated Mushrooms, 115, *122*
    Moroccan Carrots, *116*, 118
    Quinoa-Stuffed Acorn Squash with Cranberries & Feta, *110*–111
    Spinach & Artichoke Squash Casserole, *120*–121

Summer Squash Frittata, 112
White Bean & Broccolini Salad, *122*–123
Mediterranean diet
    about: this book and, 9
    advantages of, 9
    basics of, 10–11
    calorie limits and, 9
    eating more seafood, 11
    enjoying conscious indulgences, 11
    filling up on produce, 11
    meal plans and, 9
    prioritizing good-for-you fats, 10
    weight loss and, 9
    whole-grains for, 11
Mediterranean Hummus Egg Smash, *12*, 25
Metric conversion charts, 127
Minestrone, *34*–35
Mint
    Cucumber-Mint Salad, *98*–99
    Mint Pesto, 24
Mixed Greens & Herb Toss Salad, 43
Moroccan Carrots, *116*, 118
Moroccan Chicken with Preserved Lemons & Olives, 100
Mushrooms
    Beet, Mushroom & Avocado Salad, 44–45
    Chicken Cacciatore, 101
    Chicken Marsala, 96
    Marinated Mushrooms, 115, *122*

O

Old Bay Peel 'n' Eat Shrimp, *22*–23
Olive-Almond Tapenade, 117
Onion pesto, 65

P

Paella, easiest-ever, *74*, 83
Pasta and pasta alternatives
    about: benefits of pastas with legume-base flour, 55; overview of recipes, 53
    Creamy Lemon Chicken Pasta, *60*–61
    Creamy Spaghetti & Zoodles, *56*–57
    Linguine with Tuna & Chiles, 59
    Pea Pesto Pappardelle, *54*–55
    Penne with Roasted Tomatoes & Spring Onion Pesto, *64*–65
    Spring Veggie & Goat Cheese Spaghetti, *62*–63
    Tahini-Lemon Quinoa with Asparagus Ribbons, *72*–73
    Tomato-Basil Gnocchi, *52*, 58
Peas
    Greek Yellow Split Pea Dip, 18
    Lemony Asparagus, Beans & Peas, 114
    Pea Pesto Pappardelle, *54*–55
Peppers
    Grilled Veggies with Honey-Thyme Vinaigrette, *108*, 119

Honey-Soy-Glazed Salmon with Peppers, 78
Pesto
    Arugula Pesto, 19
    Homemade Pesto, 91
    Mint Pesto, 24
    Pea Pesto, 55
    Spring Onion Pesto, 65
Pizza, grilled, *16*–17
Plums, in Chicken & Red Plum Salad, 88
Pomegranate-Honey-Glazed Chicken & Squash, *104*–105
Potatoes
    about: overview of recipes, 53
    Creamy Basil Potato Salad, 66
    Crispy Smashed Potatoes with Caper Gremolata, 70
    Spanish Potato Omelet, 67
    Spicy Italian Mussels & "Frites," *14*–15
    Spinach & Gruyère Potato Casserole, *68*–69
    Spring Minestrone, *34*–35

Q

Quinoa
    Chicken Quinoa Bowls, 106
    Quinoa-Stuffed Acorn Squash with Cranberries & Feta, *110*–111
    Tahini-Lemon Quinoa with Asparagus Ribbons, *72*–73

R

Radicchio Salad with Roasted Fennel & Shrimp, 48
Rice
    Easiest-Ever Paella, *74*, 83
    Honey-Soy-Glazed Salmon with Peppers, 78
Roasted Artichokes with Caesar Dip, *28*–29
Roasted Baby Vine Tomato Grilled Chicken, 92
Roasted Cumin Shrimp & Asparagus, *86*–87

S

Salads
    about: overview of soups and, 33
    Beet, Mushroom & Avocado Salad, *44*–45
    Chicken & Red Plum Salad, 88
    Creamy Basil Potato Salad, 66
    Cucumber-Mint Salad, *98*–99
    Feta-Dill Greek Caesar, *32*, 49
    Green Goddess Carrot Salad, *46*–47
    Heirloom Tomato Salad, 113, *122*
    Kale & Roasted Cauliflower Salad, *50*–51
    Lentil Salad, 79
    Mixed Greens & Herb Toss Salad, 43
    Radicchio Salad with Roasted Fennel & Shrimp, 48
    White Bean & Broccolini Salad, *122*–123

Salmon. *See* Seafood main dishes
Sauces, dips, and spreads
  Almond-Pepper Vinaigrette, 27
  Arugula Pesto, 19
  Caesar Dip, 29
  Caper Gremolata, 70
  Greek Yellow Split Pea Dip, 18
  Green Goddess Dressing, 47
  Homemade Pesto, 91
  Honey-Thyme Vinaigrette, 119
  Mint Pesto, 24
  Olive-Almond Tapenade, 117
  Pea Pesto, 55
  Spring Onion Pesto, 65
Seafood
  about: eating more for Mediterranean diet, 11; nutritional benefits, 11; prepping mussels, 15
  Crispy Cod Cakes with Almond-Pepper Vinaigrette, *26–27*
  Linguine with Tuna & Chiles, 59
  Old Bay Peel 'n' Eat Shrimp, *22–23*
  Radicchio Salad with Roasted Fennel & Shrimp, 48
  Spicy Italian Mussels & "Frites," *14–15*
Seafood main dishes
  about: overview of recipes, 75
  Easiest-Ever Paella, *74*, 83
  Honey-Ginger Cedar Plank Salmon, *76–77*
  Honey-Soy-Glazed Salmon with Peppers, 78
  Roasted Cumin Shrimp & Asparagus, *86–87*
  Seared Salmon with Lentil Salad, 79
  Shrimp Packets with Kale Couscous, *84–85*
  Soy-Glazed Cod & Bok Choy, *80–81*
  Zesty Lemon-Herb Baked Flounder, 82
Shakshuka, plum tomato and eggplant, *30–31*
Sheet Pan Chickpea Chicken, *94–95*
Shrimp. *See* Seafood references
Skewers. *See* Kebabs/skewers
Skillet Lemon Chicken with Artichokes, *102–103*

Skillet Pesto Chicken & Beans, *90–91*
Smoky Vegan Black Bean Soup, *40–41*
Soups
  about: overview of salads and, 33
  Butternut Squash & White Bean Soup, *36–37*
  Cauliflower Soup, 38
  Lemon-Dill Chicken Meatball Soup, 39
  Smoky Vegan Black Bean Soup, *40–41*
  Spring Minestrone, *34–35*
  Winter Squash & Lentil Stew, 42
Souvlaki, lamb, *98–99*
Soy-Glazed Cod & Bok Choy, *80–81*
Spaghetti. *See* Pasta and pasta alternatives
Spanish Potato Omelet, 67
Spicy Italian Mussels & "Frites," *14–15*
Spinach & Artichoke Squash Casserole, *120–121*
Spinach & Gruyère Potato Casserole, *68–69*
Spring Veggie & Goat Cheese Spaghetti, *62–63*
Squash. *See also* Zucchini
  Butternut Squash & White Bean Soup, *36–37*
  Grilled Veggies with Honey-Thyme Vinaigrette, *108*, 119
  Pomegranate-Honey-Glazed Chicken & Squash, *104–105*
  Quinoa-Stuffed Acorn Squash with Cranberries & Feta, *110–111*
  Spinach & Artichoke Squash Casserole, *120–121*
  Summer Squash Frittata, 112
  Winter Squash & Lentil Stew, 42
Summer Squash Frittata, 112
Swordfish Kebabs with Mint Pesto, 24

T
Tahini-Lemon Quinoa with Asparagus Ribbons, *72–73*
Tapas and small plates, 13–31
  about: overview of, 13
  Arugula Pesto Crostini, 19
  Cherry Tomato Confit, *20–21*
  Crispy Cod Cakes with Almond-Pepper Vinaigrette, *26–27*
  Greek Yellow Split Pea Dip, 18

  Grilled Leek, Zucchini & Ricotta Pizza, *16–17*
  Mediterranean Hummus Egg Smash, *12*, 25
  Old Bay Peel 'n' Eat Shrimp, *22–23*
  Plum Tomato & Eggplant Shakshuka, *30–31*
  Roasted Artichokes with Caesar Dip, *28–29*
  Spicy Italian Mussels & "Frites," *14–15*
  Swordfish Kebabs with Mint Pesto, 24
Tapenade, olive-almond, 117
Tomatoes
  Cherry Tomato Casserole with White Beans & Basil, 71
  Cherry Tomato Confit, *20–21*
  Heirloom Tomato Salad, 113, *122*
  Penne with Roasted Tomatoes & Spring Onion Pesto, *64–65*
  Plum Tomato & Eggplant Shakshuka, *30–31*
  Roasted Baby Vine Tomato Grilled Chicken, 92
  Tomato-Basil Gnocchi, *52*, 58

V
Vegetables. *See also specific vegetables*
  about: importance for Mediterranean diet, 11
  Grilled Veggies with Honey-Thyme Vinaigrette, *108*, 119
  Spring Veggie & Goat Cheese Spaghetti, *62–63*

W
Weight loss, 9
White beans. *See* Beans and other legumes
Whole-grains, importance of, 11. *See also* Couscous; Pasta and pasta alternatives; Quinoa; Rice
Winter Squash & Lentil Stew, 42

Z
Zesty Lemon-Herb Baked Flounder, 82
Zucchini
  Creamy Spaghetti & Zoodles, *56–57*
  Grilled Leek, Zucchini & Ricotta Pizza, *16–17*
  Grilled Veggies with Honey-Thyme Vinaigrette, *108*, 119

Photography Credits

Chris Eckert/Studio D: 7

Mike Garten: cover, 2, 11 (bottom), 12, 20, 28, 32, 40, 46, 52, 62, 68, 72, 74, 76, 108, 110, 116, 122, back cover

© Pernille Loof: 8, 30

Danielle Occhiogrosso Daly: 6, 14, 16, 26, 34, 36, 44, 50, 54, 56, 60, 64, 80, 84, 86, 90, 94, 98, 102, 104, 120

© Jonny Valiant: 11 (top), 22

Metric Conversion Charts

The recipes that appear in this cookbook use the standard United States method for measuring liquid and dry or solid ingredients (teaspoons, tablespoons, and cups). The information in these charts is provided to help cooks outside the US successfully use these recipes. All equivalents are approximate.

METRIC EQUIVALENTS FOR DIFFERENT TYPES OF INGREDIENTS

STANDARD CUP	FINE POWDER (e.g., flour)	GRAIN (e.g., rice)	GRANULAR (e.g., sugar)	LIQUID SOLIDS (e.g., butter)	LIQUID (e.g., milk)
¾	105 g	113 g	143 g	150 g	180 ml
⅔	93 g	100 g	125 g	133 g	160 ml
½	70 g	75 g	95 g	100 g	120 ml
⅓	47 g	50 g	63 g	67 g	80 ml
¼	35 g	38 g	48 g	50 g	60 ml
⅛	18 g	19 g	24 g	25 g	30 ml

¼ tsp		=					1 ml
½ tsp		=					2 ml
1 tsp	=						5 ml
3 tsp	=	1 tbsp	=		½ fl oz	=	15 ml
		2 tbsp	=	⅛ cup	=	1 fl oz	=	30 ml
		4 tbsp	=	¼ cup	=	2 fl oz	=	60 ml
		5⅓ tbsp	=	⅓ cup	=	3 fl oz	=	80 ml
		8 tbsp	=	½ cup	=	4 fl oz	=	120 ml
		10⅔ tbsp	=	⅔ cup	=	5 fl oz	=	160 ml
		12 tbsp	=	¾ cup	=	6 fl oz	=	180 ml
		16 tbsp	=	1 cup	=	8 fl oz	=	240 ml
		1 pt	=	2 cups	=	16 fl oz	=	480 ml
		1 qt	=	4 cups	=	32 fl oz	=	960 ml
					33 fl oz	=	1000 ml = 1 L

USEFUL EQUIVALENTS FOR DRY INGREDIENTS BY WEIGHT

(To convert ounces to grams, multiply the number of ounces by 30.)

1 oz	=	¹⁄₁₆ lb	=	30 g
2 oz	=	¼ lb	=	120 g
4 oz	=	½ lb	=	240 g
8 oz	=	¾ lb	=	360 g
16 oz	=	1 lb	=	480 g

USEFUL EQUIVALENTS LENGTH

(To convert inches to centimeters, multiply the number of inches by 2.5.)

1 in	=			2.5 cm		
6 in	=	½ ft	=	15 cm		
12 in	=	1 ft	=	30 cm		
36 in	=	3 ft	=	1 yd	=	90 cm
40 in	=			100 cm	=	1 m

USEFUL EQUIVALENTS FOR COOKING/OVEN TEMPERATURES

	Fahrenheit	Celsius	Gas Mark
Freeze Water	32°F	0°C	
Room Temperature	68°F	20°C	
Boil Water	212°F	100°C	
Bake	325°F	160°C	3
	350°F	180°C	4
	375°F	190°C	5
	400°F	200°C	6
	425°F	220°C	7
	450°F	230°C	8
Broil			Grill

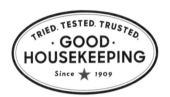

TESTED 'TIL PERFECT

Each and every recipe is developed in the Good Housekeeping Test Kitchen, where our team of culinary geniuses create, test, and continue to test recipes until they're perfect. (Even if we make the same dish ten times!)